"In *Don't Believe Everything You Feel*, author Robert Leahy provides a step-by-step guide to accepting emotions, rather than scrambling to change them; the use of adaptive, rather than unhelpful, emotional coping strategies; and an orientation to valued living. If you are experiencing emotional challenges—whether depression, or anxiety, or anger, or something else—you'll find this book to be an invaluable resource for helping to navigate those challenges."

—**David F. Tolin, PhD, ABPP**, author of *Face Your Fears*

"While animals can show all kinds of emotions that have a lot of overlap with us, humans can clearly think in a range of complex and new ways that other animals can't. While these thinking competencies make us unique, they can also drive us into anxiety and depression. In his new and deeply insightful book on the link between thinking and feeling, internationally renowned cognitive therapist Robert Leahy guides us skillfully through the minefields and problematic relations between our thoughts and feelings. He identifies clearly how our interpretations and thoughts about situations, and feelings themselves, can make us feel better or worse, engage with them, or try to avoid them. Packed with years of insightful clinical experience, this is a wonderful guide for anyone interested in the relationship between thinking and feeling, and how to get one's mind on a more balanced footing."

—**Paul Gilbert, PhD, FBPsS, OBE**, author of *Living Like Crazy* and *The Compassionate Mind*

"Leahy leads us through numerous clinical scenarios to demonstrate the emotional traps people fall into that get them stuck, and addresses nuanced aspects of emotions, including worry and rumination; envy, shame, and hopelessness; ambivalence; and effectively recognizing and responding to emotions in others.

Through numerous self-assessments and exercises, Leahy helps the reader recognize that a rich and meaningful life includes experiencing a full range of emotions, including painful ones. In explicating the centrality of emotions to the human experience, Leahy both validates his readers and invites them to keep moving forward, transcending emotion-based perceived limitations and instead using emotions to increase awareness of priorities and pursue meaningful goals."

—**Jill Rathus, PhD**, professor of psychology at LIU Post; codirector of Cognitive Behavioral Associates in Great Neck, NY; and coauthor of *DBT Skills Manual for Adolescents* and *Dialectical Behavior Therapy with Suicidal Adolescents*

"To be human is to experience a tapestry of emotions. Now, for the first time, internationally renowned author and clinical psychologist Robert Leahy offers an inspiring workbook based on his unique theory of emotion. His integration of cognitive-behavioral and acceptance perspectives is a refreshing departure from conventional therapies that take a more pathogenic view of emotion. This workbook is packed full of wisdom, guidance, intervention strategies, and step-by-step exercises and worksheets that will transform a broad range of negative and distressing emotions. Written with conviction, compassion, and encouragement, readers will find the many case examples engaging and illuminating. Leahy gently, but persuasively, guides the reader through a process of discovery and emotional transformation that enables individuals to better themselves, enrich their relationships, and experience what it means to be authentically alive."

> —**David Clark, PhD**, professor emeritus in the department of psychology
> at the University of New Brunswick

"Robert Leahy is one of most influential clinicians in the field of psychology today. His latest book, *Don't Believe Everything You Feel*, is based on the principles of cognitive behavioral therapy (CBT) as well as emotional schema therapy, and details an innovative way of coping with difficult feelings. Case examples and exercises found within illustrate how to live a full life by allowing the experience of a full range of emotions. I highly recommend this accessible and inspiring self-help book!"

> —**Sabine Wilhelm, PhD**, professor at Harvard Medical School, and chief of psychology
> at Massachusetts General Hospital

"Emotions define us as a human species. Robert Leahy's book, *Don't Believe Everything You Feel*, holds the key to understanding the secret of living a human life with its confusing experiences ranging from joy and happiness to depression and anxiety. This superb text outlines his influential emotional schema therapy approach using cognitive and behavioral principles. Written by a master clinician—one of the most influential authors and foremost leaders of CBT—this text is destined to become a classic. Clearly a must-read for any clinician, trainee, client, and anybody interested in emotions and psychotherapy."

> —**Stefan G. Hofmann, PhD**, professor in the department psychological
> and brain sciences at Boston University

Don't Believe Everything You Feel

A CBT WORKBOOK to IDENTIFY YOUR EMOTIONAL SCHEMAS and FIND FREEDOM FROM ANXIETY and DEPRESSION

Robert L. Leahy, PhD

NEW HARBINGER PUBLICATIONS, INC.

Publisher's Note

Distributed in Canada by Raincoast Books

Copyright © 2020 by Robert L. Leahy
      New Harbinger Publications, Inc.
      5674 Shattuck Avenue
      Oakland, CA 94609
      www.newharbinger.com

Daily Emotion Log from *Cognitive Therapy Techniques, 2nd Edition* by Robert Leahy. Copyright © Guildford Press 2017. Used by permission.

Cover design by Sara Christian

Acquired by Ryan Buresh

Edited by Marisa Solis

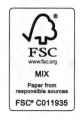 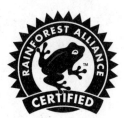

Library of Congress Cataloging-in-Publication Data on file

Printed in the United States of America

22   21   20

10   9   8   7   6   5   4   3   2   1   First Printing

To Helen

Contents

CHAPTER 1

What Are Emotions?

What is the difference between you and a robot?

Think of all the things that robots can do. They can cook your dinner, clean your floor, answer your phone, roll into a dangerous building and extract a bomb, drive your car, deliver your Amazon packages. They can beat you in chess—over and over—even if you're a world-class chess champion. They can solve just about any mathematical problem you present to them, and now robots are even used in therapy with autistic children.

So, what do you have that a robot doesn't?

Feelings.

Robots don't have the sense of anxiety, desire, sadness, anger, excitement, or loneliness that you may feel on any given day.

If you are alive, then you have feelings. And if you are conscious, you also have sensations, pain, and awareness that something is going on.

The Man Who Was Locked Inside Himself

Let me tell you a true story of someone who was completely paralyzed but still aware of what was going on around him. In 1995, the editor of the French magazine *Elle,* Jean-Dominique Bauby, suffered a stroke that resulted in a coma. Twenty days later he came to consciousness, but he was completely locked inside his body—unable to move, unable to speak—feeling helpless but aware of what was around him.

Remarkably, Bauby was still able to move his left eyelid. This led him to think about the possibility of dictating a journal about his experience. He worked out a system with his assistant that allowed him to blink when he noticed specially displayed letters of the alphabet that he wanted to "record." In the months that followed, he dictated 200,000 eye blinks, which resulted in a book about his experience: *The Diving Bell and the Butterfly.*

What strikes the reader is that every little sensation and observation he recorded had a special meaning for him. He felt sadness when he was unable to touch and feel his son, noticed the curtain moving in the breeze, heard the voices of the people who loved him, felt the loneliness on the days when there were no visitors. Bauby recalled memories of friends, travels, and smells of his experiences many years ago.

Because of impairment to his hearing, Bauby noticed the feelings he had as he heard butterflies in his head. Every moment seemed to capture a sensation, a perception, a feeling, and a meaning. He may have felt trapped in a diving bell, but he knew that he was alive, wanting to reach out, wanting to touch the people, the curtains, the bed sheets, the world "outside."

Two days after the book was published he died of pneumonia.

But even locked inside, even just blinking one eye, even being fed through a tube in his stomach, Bauby was not a robot. He was alive. And we can imagine ourselves trapped inside, unable to move, but still aware, still having the emotions that make us alive, still yearning, and still feeling lost. We feel a sense of connection and obligation to any living creature that is capable of feeling pain.

Feeling is living.

What Are Emotions?

Emotions are feelings that have meanings for us. Examples of emotions include sadness, anxiety, loneliness, anger, hopelessness, joy, ambivalence, jealousy, and resentment. We often confuse emotions with *thoughts*. However, thoughts are typically statements or beliefs about facts ("He's a loser"), while emotions are typically feelings (such as irritability) that we have about the thought. For example, you might say that you *think* things won't work out (which is a prediction) but you might not actually *feel* hopeless (since you don't care). You might *think* your former partner is involved with someone else, but you might not *feel* jealous because you have moved on. And you might *think* you will be spending the entire weekend alone, but you might not *feel* lonely.

Thoughts are not the opposite of feelings—they are different from feelings. A thought ("I am a loser") can lead to a feeling (sadness). And a feeling (sadness) can also lead to a thought ("I will always be alone").

One way to tell the difference between a thought and a feeling is to ask if a thought is true or false. For example, you can ask yourself, "Okay, is it true that he's *really* a loser? Maybe he's not totally a loser." You might be wrong about your original thought—or right. A thought can be true or false. But it would make no sense to ask if your emotions are true or false. Would you say, "I feel irritated. Is it true that I feel irritated?" Of course you feel irritated. There's no question about it. When you have a feeling, your body is telling you the truth—unless you are consciously lying to yourself.

As just mentioned, thoughts can lead to feelings; for example, the thought "He's a loser" can lead to a range of feelings, including anger, anxiety, sadness or even indifference. And feelings can lead to thoughts; for example, when you are feeling angry, perhaps you start thinking everyone around you is in your way, disrespectful, and hostile.

And we can have thoughts about our feelings. For example, you might have the thought that your loneliness will go on forever. Or that you must be weak to feel lonely. Or that your loneliness reflects how much you value being with your partner.

You can also have feelings about your feelings. You might feel embarrassed that you feel lonely, or you might feel anxious about your loneliness.

So, thoughts are different from feelings, and thoughts and feelings can influence each other, and you can have thoughts about your feelings. Take a look at Figure 1.1 to see if this makes sense.

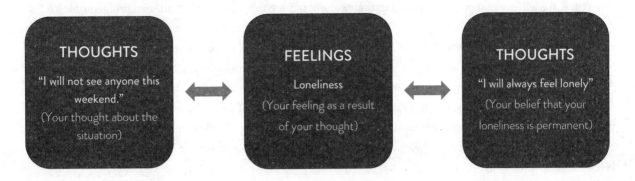

Figure 1.1

Remember how I said that we can also have feelings about our thoughts and feelings about our feelings? For example, we may feel lonely, and then we may think that we will always be alone, and then we may think that our loneliness will go on forever (Figure 1.2). In other words, we can have a thought about the emotion of loneliness, such as "My loneliness is permanent" or "Other people don't feel as lonely" or "My loneliness is out of control" or "I'm weak because I have lonely feelings." In Figure 1.2 you can see how these thoughts about our feelings lead to new feelings that may be even more disturbing than our initial feeling. and then we may feel hopeless about our loneliness (Figure 1.2).

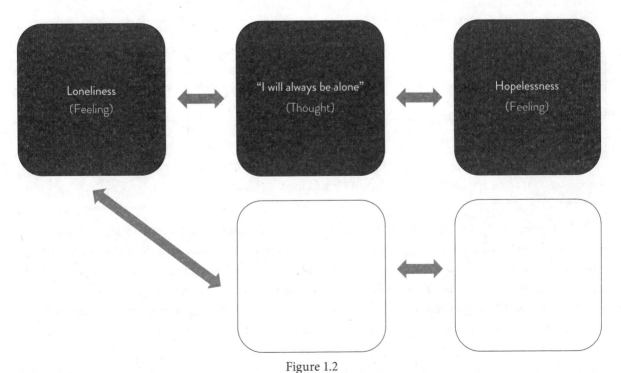

Figure 1.2

Some of us are afraid of our feelings, feel confused when we feel anxious, or feel guilty or ashamed when we feel angry. We will see that our feelings and thoughts about our feelings can create additional problems for us. For example, if you feel anxious about your anxiety, then your anxiety will escalate to even more anxiety. If you think that your anxiety is out of control and will last forever, then you will feel more anxious.

On the other hand, if you accept your anxiety, your anxiety may calm down on its own. If you say to yourself, "I notice that I am feeling anxious right now, and I accept that as an experience for this moment," you may be less anxious about your anxiety. In this book, you will learn a wide range of techniques and strategies for accepting, changing, and using your unpleasant emotions—so you don't have to be afraid of them.

Take a look at the worksheet below and check the box that correctly identifies the example in the left column—is it a thought or a feeling?

Which Are Thoughts and Which Are Feelings?

Example	Thought	Feeling
1. I will fail the exam.		
2. I am lonely.		
3. I will never find a partner.		
4. I made a stupid mistake.		
5. I am so sad I can't stand it.		
6. She is smarter than I am.		
7. I am so angry right now.		

Answers: 1, 3, 4, and 6 are thoughts, and 2, 5, and 7 are feelings.

Let's continue looking at the differences between thoughts and feelings using a relationship example. If you say, "I feel jealous," you are expressing an emotion. But if you say, "My partner finds him attractive," that is a thought. Do they sound the same? Well, if they do, maybe this can help: You can believe that your partner finds someone attractive, but you can feel any number of ways, such as ambivalent, aroused, or angry.

Let's take another comparison. "Tom was rude to me" is a thought. It's a thought *about an emotion* that you believe Tom has. It might be true that Tom was rude to you. Or it might not be true that he was rude. Maybe Tom was having a headache. But even if you thought he was rude you might not care (emotion). Just because you think that Tom is rude to you doesn't mean that you automatically have the emotion of anger. It has to *matter* to you that Tom is rude—you have to be concerned about it. You have to give some meaning to his behavior for it to make you feel an emotion. You might also have another thought that does give meaning to Tom's rudeness: "I can't stand it when someone is rude to me" or "I should be angry at people who are rude to me." These thoughts can make you angry or anxious.

So, let's put together what we know about thoughts and feelings. Let's look at Figure 1.3.

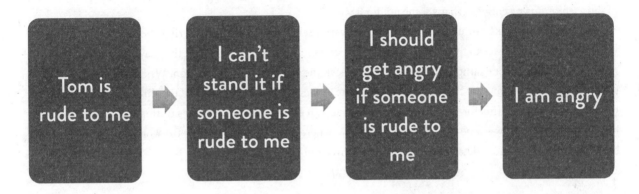

Figure 1.3

Just because someone is rude to you (let's call it a "fact") doesn't mean you have to feel angry. You might not care what Tom does or think, you might believe that you can still do everything you want to do even if someone is rude, you might think that Tom has his own problems and that he might be having a bad day, you might not take it personally. Let's see what that looks like.

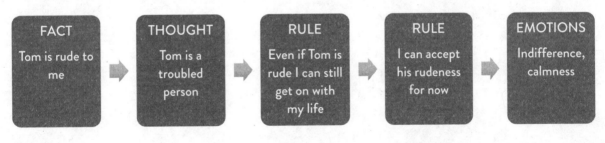

Figure 1.4

So, we can see that a fact (Tom is rude) and a thought (I can't stand it if he is rude) can lead to an emotion. But facts and thoughts don't always lead to the same emotion. Because there may be another thought—*a rule*—that makes the fact and thought a problem for us. And that rule is "I can't stand it when Tom is rude to me" or "I can't accept his rudeness."

In this book, you will see how your thoughts lead to your emotions, escalate your emotions, and can make you anxious, angry, or sad. And you will also see how you can change these thoughts and your rules so that you are not living a life on an emotional roller coaster.

Which Emotions Do You Have?

All of us have emotions, but some of us have a hard time noticing them, labeling them, and remembering them. Most of the time an emotion seems so automatic and transient that only later do you notice and label it. Let's see if you can remember having any of the emotions listed on the worksheet that follows. Have you experienced some of those emotions recently? Perhaps some not for a while?

Now, let's see if you can use the worksheet to keep track of your emotions during the next week. Begin by writing the day of the week at the top. Then note which emotions you experienced that day by checking the box next to the emotion. For example, if you felt afraid, check the box next to that emotion. When you are finished for the day, go back and circle the three emotions that were the most difficult for you and the three emotions that were the most pleasant. Do this for the next seven days. You can access additional copies of this worksheet from this book's website, http://www.newharbinger.com/44802, where you'll find other helpful worksheets (see the very back of this book for more details on accessing these free online accessories).

Daily Emotion Log

Day: _____

- ☐ Active
- ☐ Afraid
- ☐ Alert
- ☐ Angry
- ☐ Anxious
- ☐ Ashamed
- ☐ Awed
- ☐ Bored
- ☐ Challenged
- ☐ Compassionate
- ☐ Confident
- ☐ Curious
- ☐ Courageous
- ☐ Determined
- ☐ Disappointed
- ☐ Distressed
- ☐ Distrustful

- ☐ Eager
- ☐ Embarrassed
- ☐ Envious
- ☐ Excited
- ☐ Frustrated
- ☐ Guilty
- ☐ Helpless
- ☐ Hopeless
- ☐ Hostile
- ☐ Hurt
- ☐ Interested
- ☐ Inspired
- ☐ Jealous
- ☐ Lonely
- ☐ Loved
- ☐ Loving
- ☐ Overwhelmed

- ☐ Proud
- ☐ Rejected
- ☐ Sad
- ☐ Strong
- ☐ Trapped
- ☐ Vengeful
- ☐ Other emotion:

  _____

- ☐ Other emotion:

  _____

- ☐ Other emotion:

  _____

Do you notice a pattern? Are there certain events or people who trigger certain emotions? What kinds of thoughts are you having when you have these emotions?

_____

_____

_____

_____

What Triggers Your Emotions?

Sometimes we think that our emotions come out of nowhere. For instance, you might be sitting at home alone and suddenly feel a rush of anxiety come over you. Your body tenses, your heart beats rapidly. And you wonder what is going on. Perhaps you had too much coffee or you haven't eaten in seven hours. Or perhaps you were thinking about something that triggered anxiety. This happened to Dan, who was sitting at home alone on a Thursday night when he began thinking, "I have nothing planned for the weekend. None of my friends said they were available to make plans. Maybe I did something to offend them." His anxiety was triggered by thoughts of feeling rejected.

Or perhaps you are more likely to have certain emotions at certain times of the day. For example, Rebecca noticed that when she wakes in the early morning she feels sad, lethargic, a lack of energy, and hopeless about the day and her entire life.

Linda noticed that she would feel a rush of anxiety whenever she was in an elevator or a closed space—especially a toilet stall. Her thoughts were that she would get trapped in the elevator and not have enough air and no one would find her. She also thought she would accidentally get locked in the toilet stall and that she would be trapped for hours. Linda's anxiety was triggered by situations and places.

Is there a "trouble time" for you? Are there certain places, people, or situations that trigger your emotions? Recognizing your trouble times is a good step toward preparing for those moments with coping tools.

On the worksheet that follows, list your most positive and most negative emotions. For example, you might think that your most positive emotions are happiness, joy, curiosity, feeling calm, and appreciation; and you might think that your most negative emotions are anger, anxiety, sadness, and loneliness. Also list the triggers—the events, people, thoughts, or situations—that trigger your negative and positive emotions.

My Emotions and Their Triggers

My most positive emotions	_____ _____ _____ _____
My most negative emotions	_____ _____ _____ _____
Triggers for my negative emotions	_____ _____ _____ _____
Triggers for my positive emotions	_____ _____ _____ _____

Once you have completed the worksheet, review what you have written. Is there a pattern? Write down what you have noticed.

_____

_____

_____

_____

Feelings and Meanings

As we touched on earlier, feelings—such as sadness, loneliness, anger, love, and hopelessness—are tied to some meaning in our lives. For example, if you feel lonely, it likely means that human connection is important to you. If you feel angry, it probably means that being treated with respect is important to you. Feeling love means that another person is special to you. Your anxiety may mean that something important to you—your child, partner, health, or job—is in danger. Your jealousy may mean that your relationship with your partner is threatened and that this relationship is important to you. And your sadness may mean that you are feeling defeated in your attempt to get close to the person you care about—because that person has meaning for you. *We as humans have such great capacity for feelings because we give meaning to so much.*

It may be hard to put into words why you feel the way you do. When I listen to a beautiful piece of music or read an enchanting poem, I am moved—sometimes to tears. If you ask me what about it was meaningful, it would be hard for me to say. The music or words reached into my soul, touched me deeply, and afterward I struggle to find the words to capture that meaning. I imagine that you are like me in this way—at times something touches you deeply, moves you, and you feel a rush of emotion. You cannot find the words to express *why*. You just feel it. Sometimes we feel something deeply but we cannot put it into words. We are speechless.

And yet, in this workbook, we will work toward noticing and identifying your feelings, because understanding their meanings can help you live with a full range of emotions. We will look for the meanings contained in your feelings.

The Five Parts of an Emotion

Emotions have several parts to them. Often we are not fully aware of them when we experience an emotion, but they are there:

- Sensations

- Beliefs

- Goals

- Behaviors

- Interpersonal tendencies

Why are these five parts of feelings important? Because once we can identify them, we can make choices to change them. We can affect your overall emotional experience by changing any one or all of these five components. We can change your sensations, beliefs, goals, behaviors, and how you interact with people. To help you understand the role of each part, let's take anger as an example.

Sensations

When I feel angry, I notice that I have certain *sensations*: my heart is beating rapidly, I feel my body getting tense, and sounds seem to be more intense to me. But I can also have these sensations and not have the emotion of anger. For example, I can notice my heart beating rapidly because I had too much coffee.

When you have an emotion, ask yourself, "Where am I feeling it in my body?" If you are sad, for example, perhaps you feel heaviness in your chest, or you feel the energy draining out of you.

What sensations do you notice when you feel anxious, angry, and sad:

Anxious: _____

_____

Angry: _____

_____

Sad: _____

_____

Beliefs

When we have the emotion of anger, it is related to a thought or belief that we have about what is going on. This is the "meaning" part of emotion. For example, I might have the thought that the person in front of me on the highway is purposefully trying to block me from getting ahead. I might have a related thought that I can't stand this and that he is a terrible person.

What thoughts do you have when you are angry? Do you think that the other person did something to you personally? Do you think that they are a bad person?

_____

_____

Goals

My anger is about something. For example, I might be angry because I am stuck in traffic and I think I will be late. But this thought or fact might not be enough for me to feel angry. I also need to have a *goal* that is essential for me—in this case, it might be that "I need to get there on time." I am angry about traffic because it's getting in the way of my goal. Likewise, I might not be frustrated and angry if I am indifferent about being on time.

Think about your anger. Is it triggered by your concern about being listened to, treated unfairly, or blocked in achieving something? Your emotions point to your goals.

_____

_____

Behaviors

We also have a tendency toward some behavior related to the emotion. In the case of anger, I might want to attack (punch that driver in the face). When I'm not driving, I might also clench my fists, stomp my feet, throw things, or pace.

Look at your own anger. What do you do when you get angry? Do you tense up and pace around?

_____

_____

Interpersonal Tendencies

Many emotions have an interpersonal component. We may feel inclined to say something, seek out reassurance, clutch onto someone, or avoid people. For example, I might feel inclined to tell the driver that he is rude and I can't stand it, because I'm angry. When I am feeling anxious, I might turn to a close friend and seek reassurance. When I am sad and feel hopeless, I might isolate myself from others because I believe I will be a burden.

What do you do interpersonally when you have an intense emotion? Do you complain, withdraw, or seek reassurance?

_____

_____

To recap, when we first notice an emotion, we are aware of the sensations of that emotion. For example, we may first notice sadness when we feel heaviness in our chest or anxiety when we notice our heart rate is rising. Those sensations tell us that something is going on. But sensations are not the same as an emotion. For example,

I am on my third cup of coffee this morning and I just worked out. My heart rate is a little high. Am I anxious? No. I am simply feeling the residual effects of the running I did and the coffee I am drinking. This is simply *arousal*. I am not anxious about anything in particular; I am simply aroused.

But if I were someone prone to having panic disorder, I might think, "I'm having a heart attack!" I might interpret those sensations as a sign that something bad is about to happen. So, sometimes we misinterpret our sensations as a sign of something other than simply arousal. Is this familiar to you?

When we can identify the five parts of an emotion, we can target them for change. For example, I can decrease the arousal or *sensations* by practicing relaxation, mindful meditation, or other calming techniques. I can change my *beliefs* about what is going on so that I don't take the driver blocking me personally, put it in perspective as not as important, or recognize that it is temporary. I can change my *goals* by deciding to focus on something different. For example, rather than focus on getting to work on time, I can focus on listening to the radio. I can change the *behavior* that I engage in to something rewarding. And I can change the *interpersonal* actions I have with people to something that is less reactive and instead more productive.

None of this will be easy. None of it may come naturally. But all of it is important.

Now let's look at the five parts of loneliness. If you have had difficulties with loneliness, you may recognize yourself in some or all of this. Each of the five parts of loneliness can either increase or decrease your loneliness.

The Five Parts of Feeling

Loneliness

Sensations	Beliefs	Goals	Behaviors	Interpersonal Tendencies
Heavy feeling in my body	I will always be alone	To feel connected	Withdraw from others	Seek out support
Feeling empty inside	No one cares about me	To feel cared about	Lie on the couch watching movies	Contact a friend

Now let's take a look at an emotion that you might have at times—one that bothers you. Perhaps it is anxiety, sadness, anger, hopelessness, jealousy, envy, resentment, or boredom. On the following worksheet, choose one emotion and write it down in the blank space at the top. Next, write down the physical sensations that you feel in your body, such as tiredness, emptiness, muscle tension, or a rapid heartbeat. Then, write down the beliefs (thoughts) that you have when you feel this emotion; for sadness it might be "I will never be happy" or "I think that people don't want to be with me." Next, write out the goal or focus that is your concern. Finally, note how you interact with other people when feeling this emotion, such as complaining, seeking reassurance, avoidance, or seeking out company.

The Five Parts of My Emotion

The Emotion That Concerns Me: _____

Sensations	Beliefs	Goals	Behaviors	Interpersonal Tendencies

Your emotions have many parts to them. Noticing each one can help you cope better with them when they occur. I encourage you to repeat this exercise for as many emotions as you'd like to explore; you can download additional copies from http://www.newharbinger.com/44802. To reiterate, the more you are able to notice the parts of your emotions, the better success you will have at living with your full range of feelings.

What You Will Learn in This Book

Now that we know what emotions are—and how they may differ from thoughts but are also affected by them—let's look at what you will learn in this workbook. You will learn to:

Become familiar with your emotions. The purpose in writing this book is to help you understand your emotions, help you think about your emotions in more useful ways, and assist you in coping with your emotions.

Respect your feelings. You will learn how important it is to own your feelings, validate yourself, and show some compassion toward yourself.

Understand that the way you think about your emotions can make matters better or worse. Your beliefs about emotions are what I call *emotional schemas*, or *emotion beliefs*. These include your ideas that your emotions will go on indefinitely, are out of control, are dangerous, don't make sense, are different from the emotions of other people, or are shameful. You may have learned these beliefs growing up or from how other people have responded to you, but these beliefs may keep you stuck. The good news is that we can consider other ways of thinking about and responding to your emotions.

Live a full life by experiencing a full range of emotions. The reality of your life is that you cannot always be happy, you cannot avoid disappointment, and you cannot escape the agony that we all share at times. The goal is to live a life as fully, as open, and as enriched as possible—which may sometimes include the emotions that you don't like having. My approach to living a life that involves a full range of emotions—including painful and confusing feelings—is called *emotional schema therapy*. You will learn how *to normalize what seems abnormal* and *build a life large enough to include whatever disappointments* come along. Rather than expect *emotional perfectionism,* you will learn how to succeed with imperfection, how to use discomfort constructively, and how to do what you don't want to do. The message is not to *feel good*—it is the capacity to *feel everything*.

Understand that emotions are temporary. While strong emotions seem to last forever, they are temporary—even if they are frightening at times.

Realize that having a feeling is not the same thing as acting on a feeling. We will examine your shame and guilt about your feelings, and how moralistic views of emotions make it difficult to live with the very human—*all too human*—qualities that we all share. None of us is a saint, we are all fallen angels, all capable of just about anything. You will learn that emotions are not the same thing as actions or moral choices.

Make sense of your emotions. You may sometimes think that your emotions do not make sense, and this thought may lead to more shame, isolation, and rumination. But you will see that even emotions such as envy, resentment, hopelessness, and jealousy can be adaptive at times. The key is making sense of them and finding the right balance.

Not fear your feelings. You may fear your feelings because you think that they are out of control and that something terrible will happen. You might be afraid of acting on these feelings, harming yourself, going insane, or having a medical catastrophe. You will learn techniques to cope with the sense that everything is escalating.

Learn to normalize conflicting and ambivalent feelings. You may have the belief that you should only feel one way about yourself, others, or your experiences. But you will learn that having mixed feelings, or feeling ambivalent about things, does not mean you cannot make choices. In fact, ambivalence can be seen as a richness and reality of feelings rather than confusion. Making room for conflicting feelings can help you ruminate less, make helpful choices, and live with the complexity of a real life.

See how your emotions reflect your underlying values. Your character and your personal goals imbue your feelings. If you were a shallow, superficial person, things wouldn't matter to you—but you are not shallow. You are not a robot, you are not an empty person. Even if life is a roller coaster at times, you may still be able to slow it down and even direct it toward what you value. The emotions will come along for the ride.

Better connect with people important to you. We will review the problematic beliefs of and responses to the emotions of other people. You will learn how to connect in a meaningful and compassionate way to those important to you.

Develop adaptive strategies to cope with emotions. You will learn skills to help you live with a full range of feelings rather than believe that you need to get rid of those feelings. You will find out how to embrace painful emotions without getting hijacked, observe and accept emotions while coping more effectively, and move toward the life you want while also realizing that disappointment, frustration, and even unfairness will be part of that journey. The goal is to live a *real life*—not aim for a life without negative feelings. The goal is *enrichment, openness, and balance*—not emotional perfectionism, cynicism, or disillusionment.

You may say at times, "This is hard for me." But I hope that you can also learn to say, "I am the person who does the hard things." As you learn to notice, accept, and live with all the noise in your life, you will be able to overcome your fear of feeling. And then your life will be one that is more complete.

Take-Home Points

◆ Feelings mean that you are alive.

◆ Thoughts and feelings are different.

◆ Thoughts can lead to feelings and feelings can lead to thoughts.

◆ Keep track of your emotions and notice the most unpleasant and pleasant.

◆ Keep track of what triggers your emotions.

◆ Emotions have five parts: sensations, beliefs, goals, behaviors, and interpersonal tendencies.

◆ Each one of these five parts of your feelings can be a target for change.

CHAPTER 2

Validating Your Feelings

The first sound that a newborn will utter is a cry. It is as if we are born with a sense of being startled, disturbed, overwhelmed. Our tiny voice pierces whatever silence there is to call out to those around us: "Pick me up! Comfort me!" When a child cries, it is reaching out to anyone, hoping that someone will hear their pain, hoping that someone will touch them, hold them, listen to them, soothe them. There is nothing more lonely than crying alone where no one can hear you, where no one can connect with you. *We are not taught to cry, we are born to cry.*

This is universal. In one study, 684 mothers from a wide range of countries were observed for an hour responding to their baby's crying (Bornstein et al. 2017). Regardless of the mothers' nationalities, the responses were very similar: to pick up the baby, soothe them, and talk to them. MRIs of the mothers' brain indicated that the same brain regions were activated—regions associated with movement, speaking, and processing language.

In other research, scientists found that women were more likely to become alert and responsive to the crying, while men were more likely to continue in "mind wandering"—that is, not being fully attentive (De Pisapia et al. 2013). Indeed, there was no difference between experienced and inexperienced parents, suggesting that this difference is largely innate.

Research shows that mothers from many different species not only respond to crying but are able to distinguish different kinds of crying, including those of hunger, isolation, and danger (Lingle et al. 2012). Crying and our response to crying are tied to evolutionary adaptation; infants whose mothers responded rapidly to crying were more likely to grow up and give birth to babies who survived.

This behavior is explained by *attachment theory,* an idea first developed fifty years ago by British psychiatrist John Bowlby. He proposed that there is an inborn "system" of attachment that creates an almost impenetrable bond between parent (mainly mothers) and their infants. The bond is characterized by the mother's (or father's) quick response to pick up the infant, comfort the infant, and protect the infant when they cry. And yet, the child is inclined to protest, follow, or cry when a parent leaves. Why is this bond adaptive for survival? If there is no response to crying, then the child is less likely to get food when hungry, less likely to be rescued from danger, and less likely to be found when lost. This attachment bond is so powerful that parents may even risk their own safety to protect, save, and care for their infant.

Many of our emotions cry out for comfort, soothing, understanding, and caring. The infant within us needs to be understood, to have a safe place to express and share feelings. So, when we cry out, we are in emotional pain. When we are lonely, we are resurrecting that most basic, earliest system of attachment. It is as if we need to be heard, comforted, understood, protected, and connected with someone.

Joanne's Story

Joanne came to see me because of her depression after a breakup. We discovered that her depressive episodes went back to her adolescence, when she felt unloved, unwanted, and alone. She had a history of dead-end relationships with men who treated her poorly, who seemed at first to be strong and attentive but who ended up showing their narcissism by being unfaithful and unloving. She apologized to me for her "neediness," telling me she knew she should be "stronger." It's almost as if she believed she didn't have a right to be unhappy, as if her unhappiness was a burden to me.

After a few months of sessions, she said, "I think I must be losing control. I was in a movie theater and I began crying. I couldn't stop. I don't have any control over my feelings."

I asked her what the movie was, and she said, "It's the one with Mel Gibson, *We Were Soldiers.*"

The movie is about an army lieutenant who leads his troops into combat in Vietnam. I asked her what she cried about.

"You know, there is that scene when he is saying good-bye to his family. He is kissing his wife and touching his children. And I knew he would never see them again. I felt I couldn't stop crying. I lost control."

"And why does it bother you that you cried in the theater?"

"I'm an adult. I should have more control."

This struck me as a sad belief about her crying—to feel ashamed, out of control. I know that there are times when tears come to me in public places. There are times I cry in a movie, even delivering a lecture. Why does it bother her?

"Joanne, where did you learn that crying was such a shameful thing to do?"

"I remember when I was fifteen visiting my father. My parents were divorced and I didn't have a good relationship with my father. I remember talking to him about my depression, my loneliness, and I began crying. And he said to me, 'Stop crying. You are trying to manipulate me.'"

"What happened then?"

Joanne said quietly, "That night I tried to kill myself."

"If you were the director of the movie and you saw someone sitting there crying at that scene, what would you think?"

Joanne looked at me puzzled, confused. Not knowing what the right answer was, she said, "I don't know."

"I think the director would say, 'She *got* that scene. She gets it. She is my audience.'"

"I guess that's true. Yeah, I can't imagine saying good-bye to my kids. I can't imagine it." She looked down, tears in her eyes, as her voice softened, trailed off.

"I have seen how you respond when one of your children calls you while we are in session. I see how you take the time to be there for them. You don't ever want them to cry alone."

Joanne is not the only person to feel this way. Perhaps someone told you not to cry, snap out of it, get yourself together. Perhaps you were made to think that your crying was something to be ashamed of.

What were the messages you got when you were a kid? Who did you feel comfortable crying in front of?
Who did you avoid crying in front of? How did this make you feel?

_____

_____

_____

_____

_____

_____

_____

_____

_____

Think about the messages that you may have gotten about crying. Do any of these comments sound familiar?

☐   Stop crying.

☐   Get control of yourself.

☐   Don't take it so badly.

☐   You'll get over it.

☐   Your crying is upsetting me.

☐   Don't act like a child.

Or

☐   Silence

Rachel's Story

Rachel came to see me with a history of a suicide attempt, cocaine abuse, alcohol abuse, self-cutting, depression, and a string of self-defeating relationships. In her first session with me she had a superficial smile on her face as she recounted what seemed like one tragedy after another. She said, "Maybe you can teach me a *few tricks* to handle my insomnia. Otherwise, things are fine."

I asked her why she presented with such a superficial, self-denying style.

"In my family we always had to look good, sound good. Being depressed was a sign of weakness. You would be humiliated. So we all had to look good."

"I guess that is why you trivialize your own problems," I said.

Later Rachel shared with me that when she was sixteen and in Europe on vacation, her boyfriend broke up with her over the phone. The night she returned home, Rachel took an overdose of pills and became sick. Her mother told her that she must have jet lag and that she would get over it.

There was never anyone who Rachel could cry in front of. Including her mother, including me. I asked her about this.

"Actually, I used to be able to cry in front of my cat. I would talk to her, she seemed to understand, I would cry. I would hold her... I think I need to get a cat."

Over the course of our many months of work together, Rachel improved dramatically. She cut back on her drinking, stopped using cocaine, became more assertive in her relationships with men, and became a lot less depressed. A year later, she met a guy who seemed decent, but she began to sabotage the relationship. I asked her why she would want to spoil a good relationship.

"I'm afraid," Rachel replied. "I want to reject him before he rejects me."

"Maybe you could love each other rather than reject each other," I offered.

The relationship continued, and she went back and forth testing him, testing herself. After many more months, things seemed to have improved remarkably. She seemed genuinely happy. I asked her what was the most important thing that helped her.

She looked at me with a wry smile and said, "I got a cat."

When you were a child or adolescent, how did your parents respond to you when you cried? Who would you go to for support—and who would you avoid? Why?

_____

_____

_____

_____

What Is Validation?

When someone is upset, we can have a range of responses to their feelings. We can ignore them entirely and remain silent. We can tell them to stop feeling that way, to snap out of it. We can tell them it's not as bad as it seems. We can make fun of them, ridicule them, call them names.

You know that none of those responses works. They only make things worse. That's because each of these responses tells the person that their feelings are not valid, not legitimate, that they don't have a right to those feelings, that their feelings don't make sense.

This person is now all alone, and they know that you don't have room for their feelings, don't want to hear them, might even be annoyed with them. So this person is by themself, isolated, afraid, confused, and feeling sad, angry, or desperate. They have no one to reach out to. They have no connection. There is no one who hears them cry, no one who cares enough.

You know this person, because at times you may have been this person.

Validation is finding the truth in the feeling that someone has. It is respecting the moment. It is understanding what those feelings are, helping the person elaborate and expand them, giving a sympathetic and compassionate ear for the feelings that the person has. Here is what a good validating response sounds like for someone going through a breakup:

"I am here for you. Tell me how you feel. What is going on? It sounds like you are feeling sad. I can see those are hard feelings for you, but I think that they are feelings a lot of us have when losing someone we love, someone we felt connected to. I wonder if there are other feelings that you are having right now. Are you feeling confused, lonely, or hopeless? Yes, I can see that those feelings are real—they make sense in this moment. You feel these things deeply because things matter to you, because a relationship is important to you. That is the kind of person you are, someone who connects, someone others connect to. I think we need to respect those feelings right now, those are your feelings, those are real, those are feelings that matter to you, and they matter to me, too. And I realize that whatever I say, however I try to be supportive right now, it may be that whatever I try to do to care for you may not change the way you feel at this moment."

Let's summarize the different elements of a validating and caring response to someone's feelings.

- **Encourage expression.** You encourage the other person to tell you about what they're thinking and feeling: "I want to hear what you are feeling" and "Tell me what you are going through." This is like saying, "I am here for you and I hear you now." Everyone wants to be heard. Validating means listening and wanting to hear what the person has to say.

- **Reflect the pain and suffering.** You understand and reflect the pain that the other person is going through. You say, "I can see that you are sad about this" or "I can understand that you are feeling angry." Their crying out is heard.

- **Make sense of the feeling.** Not only do you encourage the person to express what they feel, you also understand how this makes sense to them at the moment. You might say, "I can see why you feel angry" or "I can see why you might feel discouraged" or "I understand that what you are going through is hard for you because of what happened."

- **Normalize the pain.** You can do this by reflecting the universal experience. You might say, "Other people feel this way" or "This is difficult for a lot of us at times." If true, you might even say, "I know what it is like for you because I have had those feelings, too." This helps the other person to feel less alone, less unique, less like some kind of outlier whose feelings are not part of the human experience.

- **Differentiate and expand emotions.** You encourage the other person to talk about a range of other feelings, not just the first feeling they are having. You might say, "Tell me what else you are feeling. What else is going on for you?" This helps expand their awareness of feelings—both positive and negative—and may help them feel better understood.

- **Link to higher values.** You can often link the way the other person feels to the values that are important to them. For example, if they are lonely, you can point to their value of feeling connected, or if they are worried about work you might link your comments to the value they place on doing a good job. You are connecting their feelings with what is important to them.

- **Respect the moment.** When you are listening and talking with the person, you are communicating that you respect the fact that at this moment this is the way they are feeling. You don't say, "Get over it" or "Move on." You might say, "I understand that this is a difficult time for you and I am here for you." In other words, *To hear the person is to be here for the person. Now* is where they are and *now* is where you are. You are both in the present moment.

- **Reflect the limits of one's validation.** You recognize that even though you are trying hard to listen, empathize, and show compassion and that you care, you also realize that this might not change anything for now. You understand the limits of what you are doing. You might say, "I know that what I say may not help right now, because I know this is a hard time." This validates the person because it reflects acceptance of their feelings in the present moment rather than insistence on changing those feelings.

Wouldn't it be nice if people responded to your feelings with this kind of validation? I wish they did. But it may be that few people are as good as they could be in connecting with you. In fact, some people may do the opposite. They may discourage you in expressing your feelings and tell you that you simply go on and on. They may tell you that they don't have time for your feelings. They may tell you that you are wrong to feel the way that you feel. They might blame you and call you names like "neurotic," "too emotional," or "out of control." All of this is invalidating and makes you feel worse.

Who Is Good at Validating You?

Although some people may not be that good at validating you, other people might be better. What can you do?

First, step back and recognize that if you are sharing feelings with someone who is critical and invalidating, then you are going to keep putting your hand in the fire and getting burned. Step away from sharing with them for now.

Second, ask yourself if there are some people who are better at validating, and share with them. Third, consider how you are sharing your feelings and ask if there might be a more skilled way to share your emotions with people. We will discuss more of this later in the section "How to Share Your Feelings" in chapter 10.

Who is good at validating you? What do they say or do that helps you feel understood and cared for?

_____

_____

_____

_____

Who is not good at validating you? What do they say or do that makes you feel invalidated?

_____

_____

_____

_____

Validating Yourself

We would like to have people who are good at validating us, but sometimes the only person we can really count on is ourself.

Let's turn to validating yourself.

REWARD YOURSELF

The great thing about rewarding yourself, validating yourself, and caring for yourself is that you are always there to do it. You can always be there to praise yourself and give credit to yourself. You don't have to wait for someone else.

One part of self-validation—of caring for yourself and recognizing the importance of how you feel—is to reward yourself as much as possible. Just as we tell parents to "catch your child being good," we can also "catch ourselves being good." For instance, in the coming week you can notice anything you do that has even the smallest amount of positive in it. For example, right now you're reading a book on how to take care of yourself. Give yourself credit for that. Or you might do some exercise or talk to a friend. Give yourself credit for that, too.

You can also validate yourself by finding the value and truth in your feelings. For example, you can validate yourself by saying, "I can listen to my feelings," "My feelings are important," and "My feelings are mine." Your feelings are real to you. Listen to your sadness and respect the fact that this is the way you are feeling right now. If it is hard for you at the present moment, acknowledge that it is hard. You can say to yourself, "I am going through a rough time. I need to be here for myself. I need to take care of myself." Take sides. *Try to be on your side.*

EXPAND THE FEELINGS THAT YOU ARE AWARE OF

You can do this by writing down all the feelings that you are aware of at the present moment. For example, Karen was feeling lonely and sad. So she wrote out her range of feelings: "I am feeling really sad, really lonely right now. I wish I had someone to talk to, but I don't. I feel discouraged. I feel anxious about my life, about ever finding someone to share my life with. I also feel angry, because I wasted so much time with dead-end relationships." There was a lot going on for her. But she could be there for herself and recognize that at that moment she was having a hard time.

Imagine yourself as your best friend. Comfort yourself and say, "I am here for you. I understand what you are going through." Normalize the way you feel by saying to yourself, "A lot of people have difficulties with loneliness, sadness, anxiety, and anger. It's part of being human. I am human just like everyone else." You are not alone in the sense that you are the only one having human feelings. You are like so many others.

Recognize that your feelings are related to your values. If you are lonely you can acknowledge and validate that your loneliness is related to a value—being connected, being with others, sharing your experience. This helps you realize that you aspire to something positive, that you are not shallow, that these are important values in your life.

REALIZE THAT SOMETIMES IT IS HARD BEING YOU

Life is not what you expect it to be at times, and you must go through disappointments, confusion, resentments, loneliness, and the inevitable conflicts and losses in relationships. You feel things deeply, you are affected by what happens in your life. What may seem like small things to some are big things to you.

Yes, it's hard being you—filled with such intense feelings, sensitive to what is around you, often plagued by thoughts of what might happen in the future. There are times when you might feel lonely—even with other people around—or times when you get angry and your anger escalates to rage. Or times when you feel a flood of anxiety and you can't quite put your finger on what it is you are anxious about.

Yes, you are fully alive with these dreadful feelings. You are perplexed and desperate trying to cope with that wide range of feelings that you are capable of. You would like to be happy all the time, but you aren't built that way—none of us is a robot.

Yes, there are times when you feel happiness, you feel love, you laugh as much as anyone, and you even feel moments of pure ecstasy about how wonderful something is that has touched you for a moment. You are capable of dancing to the poetry and music of life, even though you know that there are dark shadows and lost dreams that haunt you at times. It is the darkness and the confusion that bring you down from the heights you are capable of.

It's not easy being you. It is hard being a human being capable of feeling everything. But you are the only "you" that you have. You are stuck with you. No one else is living your life moment to moment—like you are. And it may very well be that no one fully understands what it is like for you at times.

But even when you feel alone, you are not the only one who experiences life as a roller coaster, a dark alley, a pit, a cauldron of emotional flames. No one else is really completely like you, but you are not completely different from everyone. We are all lost at times, all seeking to be found.

RECOGNIZE THAT EVERYONE HAS PROBLEMS

Sometimes you fantasize about being someone else. When you look at how wonderful everyone's life seems to be on Facebook, Instagram, or other social media, you wonder, "What is wrong with me that I am so unhappy, so lonely, so anxious?" You may think that everyone else has a happy life, great relationships, fulfilling work.

But the messages we get from social media are not real—they are advertisements for a curated life filled with positive slants, biases, posturing, and false narratives. The more time that people look at social media (like Facebook) the more depressed and envious they feel (Appel, Gerlach, and Crusius 2016; Ehrenreich and Underwood 2016). This is because social media paints a false picture of life—as if it is filled with wonderful moments, great vacations, happy and perfect marriages, and beautiful children who are always a joy to be around. Everyone is "celebrating," "grateful," and "humbled" by their privileged and perfect lives. This "humble-brag" is one of the more annoying features of the social media public advertisements of the false self.

The fact is, everyone has problems. To start with, almost 50 percent of people interviewed in national surveys has a history of a psychiatric disorder, with anxiety disorders and depression heading the list (Kessler et al. 2007). Everyone has been disappointed, everyone has people they love who die, everyone will eventually get sick, and no one feels happy all the time. The reason that we all understand the meaning of words like sad, anxious, lonely, helpless, hopeless, jealous, angry, and resentful is that at some time we all have had those feelings. We all know unhappiness. We are not a race of happy faces.

Nikki's Story

Nikki, twenty-eight, was a kind, generous, and caring person—and she felt overwhelmed with sadness, loneliness, and thoughts that she would never find a partner. At our first session, we established that she had idealized everyone she knew—everyone seemed to have a wonderful life—while she devalued her own life and her own feelings.

Then the following week Nikki came in and began our meeting with a sarcastic look on her face.

"Well, I guess I was wrong about how happy everyone is," she said smiling. "After our meeting I was walking down the street and I saw this very attractive woman in a red dress and I felt so jealous. I was thinking, 'She is so much prettier than I am, and she has that beautiful red dress. She must have a great husband. Look at me, dowdy, alone.' And then I saw two men come up from behind her, tap her on the shoulder, and tell her she was under arrest." Nicole laughed, recognizing how other people are not always what the package seems to say.

Sometimes it helps to normalize what seems abnormal to us. If we realize that suffering, disappointment, and sadness come with the territory of being fully alive, then we can count ourselves as part of the human race. We can look around us and see that we are all in this together, all struggling to make things work, all facing disappointments, all realizing that people will let us down, all knowing that we are humans filled with the capacity for love, joy, compassion, and even ecstasy—but also capable of feeling sad, helpless, anxious, and lonely.

ACKNOWLEDGE UNIVERSAL COMPASSION

Let's step away from how you are feeling and try to connect with the feelings of other people. I walk to work every day, about one mile down Third Avenue in New York City. As I walk along, I see people rushing to work, people with baby carriages, older people with walkers and canes. I see delivery people riding bicycles, a woman in a wheelchair with a cup for donations. I am looking for my morning dose of compassion—not so much to receive it but to wish it for others. Compassion can soothe, comfort, and connect us to others (Gilbert 2009).

My first encounter is watching someone with a baby stroller. I notice the loving-kindness of the mother or the nanny. I think, "She is taking care of this baby, she is giving love every day." I notice the love and I feel it in my heart. I feel their love toward each other. I then notice a delivery person on a bicycle in heavy traffic. He is likely someone who is poor, recently arrived, and this is the only job he could get. He is riding his bike in a dangerous situation to pay his bills. I feel compassion for him, I wish him well, I hope he is safe. I know that his life can be hard at times, and I reach out in my heart to hope for his happiness, for his safety, for his life to be better for him. And my heart feels it is growing, and I am more alive at this moment.

I am outside myself.

I notice a dog being taken for a walk. I see the owner, proud of her puppy, watching every move, watching the tail wag. I can see her love and care for this little guy, see that she loves her dog and that the dog loves her. And the dog is excited about every smell, about every time someone stops to say, "What a beautiful dog." I reach out with my awareness of her compassion and love, notice it, and register it in my heart.

I am collecting compassion on my way to work.

One evening, after a particularly long day, I was heading home. A few blocks into my walk I saw an elderly woman stepping uncertainly, trying to cross the street and avoid the passing cars, frail and afraid. I reached over to her and said, "Can I walk with you across the street?" She thanked me and I walked with her to the opposite corner. We exchanged names, and she said, "Thank you, Bob, for helping me. You are very kind." And I said, spontaneously, because I really meant it, "No, thank you for letting me help you. It really made me feel good to be able to help you."

Here is an exercise for you to do every day for the next week. I want you to notice any examples of kindness that you see. It could be someone pushing a baby in a stroller, someone holding the door for someone else, someone asking another person how they are, or someone walking their dog. All of these are examples of kindness. When you see the kindness, acknowledge it, imagine what it is like to give the kindness and what it is like to receive it. How do you feel when you see this kindness?

Examples of Kindness That I See

Examples of Kindness	How I Feel When I See This

Noticing kindness makes you feel more optimistic, more aware of the fact that others can be generous and compassionate. Let's imagine that you start directing some kindness toward yourself, some compassion, some support. Imagine some of the feelings that you have that concern you—sadness, loneliness, anxiety, hopelessness, envy, or anger. Now, I want you to imagine the kindest, most loving person in the world standing next to you, with their hand on your shoulder, leaning toward you and whispering the warmest most loving message they can say. What do they say?

Nikki, who thought everyone's life was better than hers, imagined a loving voice saying to her when she was lonely, "I know it is hard being lonely, hard being sad. But you are loved and you are important to me. You are a good person who really deserves happiness." Think about the warm, soothing message that you can direct toward yourself when you are feeling upset. You can be your own guardian angel.

Fill out the following worksheet. In the first column, briefly describe the situation you are in when you are having unpleasant feelings (e.g., "I am alone sitting on the couch"). In the second column, list the emotions that you are having (e.g., loneliness, sadness). In the third column, describe a kind, loving, supportive message to yourself (e.g., "You are loved," "You are a good person," "I want you to feel cared for").

Directing Kindness Toward Myself

Situation	Feelings	Kind Words Toward Myself

Take-Home Points

- Crying is part of human existence.

- We can feel comforted by others when we are suffering.

- Validation helps us realize that others care and that we are not alone.

- You can validate yourself.

- Look for examples of compassion around you—in the present and the past.

- Direct compassion toward yourself.

- Realize that every feeling you have is shared with all the human race.

- Notice acts of kindness in others.

- Direct compassion and kindness toward yourself.

CHAPTER 3

Thinking About Your Emotions

Once an emotion arises—once we are feeling sad, anxious, or angry, for example—we respond to it with our thoughts about it and our strategies to cope with it.

Let's look at how this plays out for two young men, Michael and Nate, both of whom coincidentally just broke up with their girlfriends. Each of the men had been involved for four months, and their relationships were up and down—sometimes really terrific, sometimes miserable.

Michael and Nate's Stories

Michael is a balanced guy who takes things in stride, but he's also capable of feeling the full range of emotions. When he gets the text message from Maria that she does not want him to contact her, he is immediately upset. He feels angry, anxious, confused, and sad. He had hoped that they would work things out, although he had felt ambivalent for the last two months. Initially, he feels a heavy feeling of sadness come over him. He thinks, "This is terrible" and "I can't stand this." But then he begins to realize that the sadness will be temporary. He tells himself, "It's normal to have this range of feelings. It's normal to be sad, anxious, and angry." Michael gives himself credit for being human. Although he feels sad and anxious, he is not afraid of those feelings. He doesn't think the feelings will overwhelm him, he won't go crazy.

Michael calls his friend Juan, who has always been there for him, and they get together for a couple of beers. Michael expresses the way he feels with Juan, who is a good listener and who encourages Michael to talk about his feelings. Juan tells Michael that all these feelings make sense and that he is upset because he knows that Michael wants a committed relationship and hopes to get married someday. *The loss hurts because things matter.*

After a few days, Michael is feeling somewhat better but still has waves of sadness and confusion. He goes to work, sees his friends, and continues to keep his schedule at the health club. Although he has difficulty sleeping, he realizes that this is a transition time for him and that he will get through this.

Michael is not afraid of his feelings and he doesn't feel the need to escape from them by over-drinking. He says to himself, "You have to go through it to get past it." He is willing to tolerate and accept the emotional roller coaster as he realizes that life can be difficult at times but that the difficult times change.

But Nate has a different experience when he gets the breakup text message from Nancy. He is overwhelmed with intensity. He shifts into feeling numb, almost like a zombie. He feels that this is unreal, he must be dreaming, he can't believe it. Nate then stomps around his apartment looking again and again at the text message. He groans in agony and then curses Nancy. He is filled with anger, then sadness, then confusion—like waves in a hurricane drowning him in the intensity of his feelings. He can't believe it. Nate becomes anxious that he is getting so anxious, and he fears that he will have a panic attack. He begins to tremble and thinks, "I must be going crazy." Afraid that he will lose all control and that these feelings will last forever, he punches the wall. He has to get rid of these feelings immediately. He pours himself a stiff scotch and drinks it down, hoping to get rid of these feelings.

The next day, Nate wakes and feels overwhelmed with sadness. He can't make sense of why his feelings are so intense. He thinks, "I am a grown man, why am I so weak?" He remembers his father telling him that men don't cry, and he starts to cry. Now he thinks that his crying will never stop and he becomes more anxious. "I have to stop crying," Nate says to himself.

He does have a good friend, Kevin, but he thinks that Kevin will think he is a loser for being so upset over a breakup. He feels embarrassed about his weakness. He feels overwhelmed and decides to stay home from work. He doesn't want to see anyone in his state, so he lies on the couch and turns on the television. He thinks that other men would not feel this upset, that they would be able to handle it. They would laugh it off and move on. But his sadness seems to stay, and now he thinks that he will be depressed and anxious for a long time. He dwells on how sad he feels and keeps thinking, "What is wrong with me?" He can't accept his feelings and he wants to lose himself, stop all of this feeling. He wants to feel numb.

Nate begins to loathe himself, thinking of himself as weak, out of control. He thinks, "No wonder she broke off with me. I am such a loser." He thinks that he should be strong, in control of his emotions. As he begins to cry, he thinks again, "Why am I so weak? Other men don't cry."

As he sinks deeper into his fear and rumination about his emotions, Nate becomes more depressed, helpless, and self-critical. He lacks any compassion for himself, and he drinks more to get rid of these feelings.

Emotional Schemas: Responses to Your Feelings

These two men experience the same initial emotions during the breakup: sadness, anger, anxiety, and confusion. Yet they differ in how they respond to their emotions.

Michael notices his feelings and labels them—"I am feeling sad, anxious, lonely, and discouraged." He then goes on to view his emotions as normal, not problematic, not something that he has to get rid of immediately. He is able to accept his feelings and understands that his emotions signal that something matters to him—his value of wanting a committed relationship. He also views his feelings as painful but temporary, and realizes that although he feels things intensely, the emotions won't go out of control and drive him insane. Michael is not embarrassed about his feelings, so he shares them with a trusted friend, who helps him cope. Although Michael is going through these feelings in the present moment, he believes he will get past them. And he accepts the journey along the way.

Nate's experience is very different. He has a more neurotic and problematic belief about his emotions. He believes that his emotions don't make sense, that they are problematic, and that he has to get rid of them as soon as possible. He thinks that he should be strong and in control of his feelings, and that other men do not have such strong feelings. He fears his feelings and suppresses them by drinking. Nate feels embarrassed, thinks that his feelings aren't normal, and believes others will judge him. Nate can't normalize his emotions, and in fact he has contempt for the way that he feels. He isolates himself, ruminates, avoids his friends, and doesn't go to work. Nate sinks into a depression that lasts for months.

Once an emotion arises, we respond to it from a range of beliefs and strategies. These beliefs and strategies are called *emotional schemas.* As we saw with Michael and Nate, the same situation can trigger the same feelings, but how each person responds to them is quite different. And yet, the response happens in a cycle that's identical. Take a look at Michael's Emotional Schema, then contrast it with Nate's Emotional Schema. As you can see, one deals with anxiety in a way that's problematic because it causes more problems; the other has an adaptive response to anxiety that allows for accepting the emotion and a range of other feelings at the same time, which leads to growth.

Nate's Emotional Schema

Anxiety

"This anxiety will last forever. It will go out of control."

"My anxiety doesn't make sense. I shouldn't feel this way."

I try to suppress my emotion and I fail.

I feel helpless and hopeless.

Problematic Beliefs and Responses to Emotions

I have identified fourteen problematic beliefs and responses that we have toward our emotions:

- **Invalidation** is the belief that other people don't understand or care about your feelings. Or do you believe that your friends or partner understand how your feelings make sense to you?

- **Incomprehensibility** refers to your belief that your emotions don't make sense to you, that they seem to come out of nowhere, or that you can't figure out why you are feeling so anxious or sad. Or do you believe your emotions do make sense and that there is a good reason for feeling the way you do?

- **Guilt** refers to your belief that you shouldn't have these feelings—you might think that your anger or sexual feelings are wrong to have. Or you might feel ashamed if other people knew that you had certain feelings. For example, you might feel ashamed if someone knew that you were envious of their success. Or do you see your emotions as human, natural, okay to have?

Michael's Emotional Schema

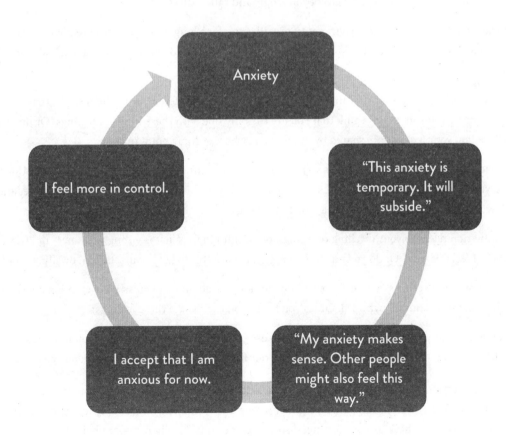

- **Simplistic view of emotion** is the belief that you should not be ambivalent about yourself or anyone else—you should only feel one way. You can't tolerate mixed feelings. Or do you think that life is complicated, so having "contradictory" feelings makes sense at times?

- **Devalued** reflects your belief that your emotions are not related to your values, that there is no valid purpose connected with your emotions. Or do you believe that painful feelings are related to important issues in relationships and the meaning of life?

- **Loss of control** beliefs reflect the thought that your strong emotions will get out of control, so you think that you have to keep them in check or they will unravel. Or do you believe that your emotions will vary in intensity but eventually become tolerable?

- **Numbness** reflects a belief that you don't experience emotions—especially strong emotions—when other people might experience these same emotions. What moves other people does not seem to affect you. Or do you notice and fully experience your feelings?

- **Overly rational** reflects an anti-emotion belief, that is, you think it is extremely important to be rational and logical, and that emotions simply get in the way. Or do you realize that not everything is rational, that there are experiences beyond logic and rationality?

- **Duration** reflects the idea that your emotions will go on for a long time, that they are not temporary. Or do you view your emotions as experiences that come and go and have a natural end in themselves?

- **Low consensus** reflects a belief that your emotions are very different from the feelings that other people have. You sometimes think that you are the only one with these kinds of feelings. Or do you believe that your feelings are shared by others everywhere at some point in time?

- **Nonacceptance** of emotions reflects your belief that you cannot tolerate or accept your emotions, that you think you need to avoid or escape them. Or do you think that you can accept, tolerate, and allow yourself to have the feelings that you are having?

- **Rumination** refers to your dwelling on things, often thinking, "What is wrong with me?" or "I can't believe I feel this way." Or do you notice an emotion but are able to keep yourself from dwelling on it?

- **Low expression** reflects your belief that you cannot talk about or express your emotions without feeling self-conscious or awkward. Or do you think you can't share these feelings?

- **Blame** refers to your belief that other people cause you to have the feelings that you have. It's their fault. Or do you take a nonjudgmental view of your feelings, neither blaming others nor yourself?

Now let's look at your emotional schema, or how you think about and respond to your emotions. We all differ in how we deal with our feelings, so there are no right or wrong answers. The goal is simply to begin to understand the unhelpful reactions you have to your feelings—so you can eventually choose more helpful responses when you're triggered.

Emotional Schema Scale

Please carefully read each common belief about emotions, which are divided by the fourteen categories of responses. Next to each statement, rate how truthfully the sentence reflects how you have dealt with your feelings during the past month, using the scale provided.

Scale:

1 = very untrue of me

2 = somewhat untrue of me

3 = slightly untrue of me

4 = slightly true of me

5 = somewhat true of me

6 = very true of me

Beliefs About Your Emotions	Response (1–6)
Invalidation	
Others do not understand and accept my feelings.	
No one really cares about my feelings.	
Incomprehensibility	
There are things about myself that I just don't understand.	
My feelings don't make sense to me.	
Guilt	
Some feelings are wrong to have.	
I feel ashamed of my feelings.	
Simplistic view of emotion	

Beliefs About Your Emotions	Response (1–6)
I like being absolutely definite about the way I feel about someone else.	
I like being absolutely definite about the way I feel about myself.	
Devalued	
My painful feelings are not related to my values.	
I do not have a clear set of values that I aspire to.	
Loss of control	
If I let myself have some of these feelings, I fear I will lose control.	
I worry that I won't be able to control my feelings.	
Numbness	
Things that bother other people don't bother me.	
I often feel numb emotionally, as if I have no feelings.	
Overly rational	
It is important for me to be reasonable and practical rather than sensitive and open to my feelings.	
I think it is important to be rational and logical in almost everything.	
Duration	
I sometimes fear that if I allow myself to have a strong feeling, it would not go away.	
Strong feelings seem to last a very long time.	

Beliefs About Your Emotions	Response (1–6)
Low consensus	
I often think that I respond with feelings that others would not have.	
I think that my feelings are different from those of other people.	
Nonacceptance of feelings	
I do not accept my feelings.	
I can't allow myself to have certain feelings.	
Rumination	
When I feel down, I sit by myself and think a lot about how bad I feel.	
I often say to myself, "What's wrong with me?"	
Low expression	
I do not believe that it is important to let myself cry in order to get my feelings out.	
I do not feel that I can express my feelings openly.	
Blame	
If other people changed, I would feel a lot better.	
Other people cause me to have unpleasant feelings.	

Now, as you look over your responses to the Emotional Schema Scale, which categories of beliefs seem to be the highest for you? Which of the categories include a response of 5 (somewhat true of me) or 6 (very true of me)? Circle the ones that are most troubling for you.

Problematic Strategies for Handling Your Feelings

All of us have unpleasant and difficult emotions at times. That is part of being human. But sometimes we try to cope with our emotions by using strategies that may make things worse. For example, when Karen felt overwhelmed by her feelings, she would binge eat or use marijuana, hoping this would help her escape from the painful feelings that plagued her. But binge eating led to gaining weight, which she tried to compensate for by vomiting and using laxatives. This made everything worse. And her reliance on marijuana seemed to rob her of her motivation to do very much of anything. She became more withdrawn.

There are a number of problematic strategies that you might use that can make things worse for you in the long run. Look at the following worksheet to determine if you use any of these.

Problematic Strategies for Coping with My Feelings

Reflect on how you have coped with your emotions during the past month. Do you use any of these strategies? Use the scale below to rate your response in the middle column. Then, in the far right column give an example of the response that you have used.

Scale:

1 = very untrue of me

2 = somewhat untrue of me

3 = slightly untrue of me

4 = slightly true of me

5 = somewhat true of me

6 = very true of me

How I Cope with My Emotions	Rate (1–6)	Example
Avoid situations		
Leave or escape from situations		
Drink alcohol		
Binge eat		
Take drugs		
Constantly ask for reassurance		

How I Cope with My Emotions	Rate (1–6)	Example
Worry about the future		
Dwell on my feelings about the past		
Blame other people		
Complain		
Engage in risky sexual behavior		
Space out on the Internet or television		
Sleep excessively		
Pull my hair or pick my skin		
Cut or harm myself		
Other:		
Other:		

Look at your responses to the strategies that you use more often and think about the effects that these strategies have on you. Are they making things better or worse?

Why Are These Strategies Problematic?

I consider these *problematic strategies* because although they may help you to momentarily reduce or eliminate an unpleasant emotion, they add another problem for you to deal with. For example, if you rely on avoidance or escape, then you are drastically limiting your experiences in life; avoidance is often the precursor to depression. If you rely on alcohol or drugs, then you may develop a dependence on these substances that will make you more prone to anxiety, depression, and interpersonal difficulties.

If you continually ask for reassurance from other people, then you will not learn to make decisions on your own, and other people may give you bad advice. If you worry about the future or dwell on the past—trying to eliminate uncertainty or figure it out—you will find yourself living in a world that often doesn't exist; you will continually focus on the negative, and you will not be able to be fully present in your current life. If you blame other people, you will add another emotion to your repertoire—anger—and this might interfere with your relationships with other people.

Complaining may give you the feeling that other people understand you, but complaining may also drive people away. Trying to deal with your feelings by relying on sexual behavior can be pleasurable and exciting at times, but you also run the risk of getting involved in relationships that add to your problems. Many of us space out on the Internet or binge on television; this can sometimes be enjoyable, but it may remove you from living a full life and may disconnect you from your friends. When you use excessive sleep to cope with unpleasant emotions, you add to your passivity and isolation, and reduce your chance to fully immerse yourself in a meaningful life; in fact, passivity, isolation, and avoidance are the hallmarks of depression.

Many people self-soothe by picking their hair or skin, or biting their nails; this can momentarily distract you from your emotions and even give a few minutes of pleasure, but you may lose your hair, damage your skin, or, if you swallow your hair or nails, cause medical problems for yourself. Sometimes you may feel so overwhelmed by your emotions that you might cut or harm yourself in some way. This, of course, is dangerous—and only adds to your belief that you are out of control.

Fortunately, you can learn a wide range of *helpful strategies* to handle your emotions. But first it is important to be honest and realistic about the unhelpful strategies so that you can begin to eliminate them.

Take-Home Points

- How we think and act when we have an emotion can make things better or worse.

- Emotional schemas are our beliefs about emotions and our strategies for coping with them.

- If you believe that your negative emotions will last indefinitely, go out of control, or don't make sense—or that you are different from everyone—then you are more likely to become anxious and depressed.

- If you believe other people have the same feelings that you have, that feelings come and go, and that you can tolerate mixed feelings, you are less likely to be upset about your feelings.

- Your negative emotions will get worse if you use problematic strategies to cope with these feelings.

- These problematic strategies include worry, avoidance, blaming, substance misuse, binge eating, and complaining.

CHAPTER 4

The Emotional Schema Approach

During the past fifteen years I have developed an approach for helping people cope with their emotions. I call it *emotional schema therapy*. I emphasize how each of us has our own theories about emotion and how to cope with them (Leahy 2015; Leahy 2018). For example, some of us believe that certain emotions are "bad," and then we feel ashamed of those feelings.

As you learned in the previous chapter, some people think it is "bad" to feel jealous or angry or lonely, while others think it's okay to have these feelings. Some believe that if we allow ourselves to have a strong emotion it will last indefinitely, incapacitate us, and cause irreparable harm; others think that a strong emotion will go away with time, so they can accept it. Problematic theories about emotions lead to problematic strategies to cope with those emotions, such as using drugs or alcohol, avoiding situations that elicit our feelings, blaming other people, dwelling on and ruminating about our experience, worrying about the future, or continually asking for reassurance.

Emotional schema therapy is not a feel-good approach to life—it's a *realistic* approach that proposes that difficult and pleasant emotions are all part of the experience of a full life. Rather than focusing on *feeling good,* we focus on the capacity to *feel everything* and grow in the process. The goal is to help you find the richness in the meaning in life—rather than taking a superficial and dismissive approach that would rob you of your capacity to feel deep feelings. You will learn to be able to accept, tolerate, and use your emotions in constructive ways—rather than fear and suppress your feelings.

The Five Principles of Emotional Schema Therapy

Many of us hold problematic beliefs about our feelings—that we should not have the feelings that we have, that other people don't have the same feelings, that our emotions are out of control, that we have to eliminate an unpleasant feeling immediately. These are problematic because they are unrealistic. Also problematic are certain strategies for coping with your emotions that make things worse.

Before we examine helpful strategies that you can start practicing today, let's take a look at the five principles of the emotional schema approach that can help you learn to live with your feelings rather than run away from or eliminate them:

- Difficult and unpleasant emotions are part of everyone's experience.

- Emotions warn us, tell us about our needs, and connect us with meaning.

- Strong emotions can lead us or mislead us.

- Beliefs about emotions can make it difficult for us to tolerate our feelings.

- Strategies for coping with our emotions can make matters better or worse.

Difficult and Unpleasant Emotions Are Part of Everyone's Experience

If you believe that you shouldn't feel anxious, then you will feel anxious about feeling anxious. If you feel guilty about feeling angry, then you will feel angry, guilty, anxious, *and* confused. And if you think you should never feel envious of someone who is doing better then you, you will have a hard time facing the inequities of daily life.

Humans have a full range of emotions that have helped us adapt to the dangers, conflicts, and demands of life in a world of scarcity and danger. Our prehistoric human ancestors contended with starvation, deprivation, threats from other humans, and dangerous animals. Life was often brutish, filled with sudden death and loss, and our emotions evolved to tell us about these dangers and to keep us on alert.

Painful and unpleasant emotions are universal. You are not alone. Everyone is capable of feeling any of the emotions that you experience. The reason we are able to talk to people about our anger, anxiety, sadness, loneliness, helplessness, and confusion is that everyone has had those experiences at some point. We are connected by our feelings.

Why is this important? It's important because knowing that you share your emotions with the rest of humanity makes you feel less different, less defective, and less alone. If we go back hundreds or even thousands of years to read literature, we learn that in the ancient Middle East 4,500 years ago an anonymous author wrote about the Heroic Gilgamesh: "He had seen everything, had experienced all emotions, from exaltation to despair, had been granted a vision into the great mystery, the secret places, the primeval days before the Flood" (Miller 2004).

We know that the classic Greek warriors in Homer's *Odyssey* and Virgil's *Aeneid* cried, felt sad, were afraid, sought revenge, and yearned to return to their homeland. Shakespeare described Othello's jealousy, Hamlet's desire for revenge, and King Lear's sense of humiliation and betrayal. We know that in every culture people grieve over the death of people they love and that men and women cry publicly. The songs that we listen to tell us about love, loss, and desire. Everywhere around us emotions call out to be heard. You are feeling your emotions because you hear what life is telling you at this moment.

Almost everyone at some point feels everything. You don't go through a full life without a full range of emotions. You are not the only one feeling angry, lonely, hopeless, helpless, ashamed, guilty, jealous, or vengeful.

How would you think and feel if you realized that everyone is capable of every feeling that you experience?

_____

_____

_____

_____

_____

Emotions Warn Us, Tell Us About Our Needs, and Connect Us with Meaning

Emotions such as fear of heights, closed spaces, and strangers tell us that there may be danger ahead. These emotions motivate us to escape or avoid. Without the intensity and sense of urgency of these emotions, our ancestors never would have survived. Fear and anger gave our ancestors a sense of urgency as they were escaping from dangerous animals and threatening humans. Just as the sensation of hunger tells us we need food, our loneliness tells us about our need for connection, our need to touch others and be touched by others.

Our anger tells us about our sense of injustice, the meaning of fairness, our desire to defend our sense of honor and decency. When we are moved by feelings of love—or feelings of loss—our emotions convey how meaningful a person or item is to us. It is virtually impossible to go through life enjoying the meaning of connection, love, and friendship without experiencing at some point feelings of loss, disappointment, and even disillusionment.

We have emotions because things matter to us, because we give meaning to our experience, because we care. Without emotions, life would be empty, robotic, and meaningless.

How do your emotions tell you about your needs, rights, and values? Give examples.

_____

_____

_____

_____

_____

Strong Emotions Can Lead Us or Mislead Us

We need our emotions to tell us what is important and help us make decisions. Our emotions can tell us that "this feels right" or "this is dangerous." But they can also can mislead us. For instance, we can conclude that something is dangerous simply because we feel anxious: "This plane is dangerous. I know because I feel anxious." This is called *emotional reasoning*, and it can lead us to think that a minor inconvenience is a catastrophe.

We can end up acting impulsively on an intense emotion and live to regret it. We can feel angry and become hostile to our partner or friend—and later realize that we had misinterpreted what was happening and acted against our long-term interests. We can feel lonely and sad, and try to lessen the pain with alcohol, drugs, or food. Later we regret it. Intensity of emotion can often be a sign that we are overreacting—that we need to step back, think things through, and consider the longer-term consequences. Feeling strongly about something is no guarantee that we are right. We could be. But we might be responding to the emotion of the moment, not to the bigger picture.

We will learn how *emotional hijacking* can lead to feeling out of control and to behaviors that we might regret. Noticing the hijack when it occurs, noticing that we are feeling overwhelmed with anger, anxiety, sadness, and hopelessness will be a good sign that we need to step back—and use the techniques described in this book.

Do you recognize yourself being hijacked? Have you said or done things when you felt overwhelmed that you later regret? You are not alone. But regret can be a useful tool to learn from your experience. *Don't waste a mistake.* Use it to correct yourself in the future—to catch yourself being hijacked and start using better tools to help yourself.

How have your strong emotions led you to say or do things that you later regret? What was the consequence?

_____

_____

_____

_____

_____

Beliefs About Emotions Can Make It Difficult for Us to Tolerate Our Feelings

If you believe your emotions will last indefinitely, then you will become anxious as soon as a strong emotion arises. If you believe that your emotions will incapacitate you, then you will immediately try to rid yourself of these feelings. In both cases, you will become anxious about your feelings, and this will spiral you into greater intensity of unwanted feelings.

If you believe that your feelings don't make sense, then you will ruminate on "Why do I feel this way?" or continually ask for reassurance from other people. If you believe that you should only feel one way about someone, then it will be difficult for you to tolerate ambivalence. You might feel guilty and ashamed about your feelings, even though your feelings may be similar to those that many others experience.

Do you have any of these beliefs about your emotions? You will learn that your beliefs about emotion can be changed. And this change can help you avoid the emotional panic that has hijacked you.

Do you believe that your emotions will last a long time, overwhelm you, or be intolerable? If so, how have your beliefs led you to think, say, or do things that you regret?

_____

_____

_____

_____

_____

Strategies for Coping with Our Emotions Can Make Matters Better or Worse

We all have our own ways of coping with difficult feelings. There are helpful and unhelpful strategies. The unhelpful strategies include avoiding anything that makes us feel uncomfortable, drinking heavily, ruminating about our feelings ("What is wrong with me?"), blaming other people, bingeing on food, spacing out on the Internet, becoming passive, and isolating ourselves.

The problem with these unhelpful coping strategies is that each of them will make things worse in the long run. You may initially feel less anxious if you drink or binge eat, but you will then have the additional problems of a hangover and feeling out of control.

Do any of these unhelpful strategies sound familiar? Again, this is part of human nature, and you need to be compassionate toward yourself when you recognize this. Your coping style has been your way to "take care" of yourself in the present moment—and now you will learn more helpful strategies to cope with your feelings. Once you have learned new ways to think about your feelings and cope with them, you will be less afraid of your feelings.

What problematic strategies have you used to cope with your feelings? How has this affected you? Have these coping strategies led to other problems for you?

_____

_____

_____

_____

_____

Six Wise Strategies

We are a consumer society, and many of us look for self-help books that will immediately make us happy and make our life easy. This is not one of those books. No, I am taking a more realistic approach to life that I think you will recognize as more authentic and more consistent with how you experience life. I am not trying to make your life easy—because I know that life is not always easy. *I want to help you live a realistic life.*

These are called *wise strategies* because they help us cope with the real world—and part of the real world is our emotions. Here they are:

- *Emotional realism*

- *Inevitable disappointments*

- *Constructive discomfort*

- *Do what you don't want to do*

- *Successful imperfection*

- *Flexible satisfaction*

Emotional Realism

Sometimes we believe that our emotions should be good, happy, easy, pleasant, and completely clear to us. This is what I call *emotional perfectionism*. It's as if we expect our life to be smooth sailing, happy faces, celebrations of everything, and always easy. That's not a life that anyone has. With the popular emphasis on feeling happy, with smiley faces staring at you from your screens, you may wonder what is wrong with you that you are not walking around with a happy smile all the time. Emotional perfectionism reflects the false belief that your emotions should be "good," "happy," and "uncomplicated." It sets you up for being unable to tolerate sadness, frustration, jealousy, or loneliness.

Emotional perfectionism makes it difficult to make decisions, because you want a guarantee that you will feel perfectly fine with your choices. You won't be able to tolerate ambivalence, tradeoffs, or frustration, and you will end up ruminating about your feelings because you think, "I can't understand why I feel this way." Emotional perfectionism gives you the unrealistic expectation that your unpleasant and difficult emotions are a sign of some deeper flaw. You think you should not feel anxious, resentful, jealous, confused, sad, or lonely. And as a result, the inevitable emotions of real life become an added burden.

I suggest a different approach. I call it *emotional realism*, which makes room for *all* emotions, helps you accept them, normalizes what seems abnormal to you, and allows you to tolerate the difficult feelings that are part of everyone's life.

How would it help you to give up on your emotional perfectionism and embrace emotional realism? What would change for you?

_____

_____

_____

_____

_____

Inevitable Disappointments

Related to emotional realism is the recognition that you will be disappointed at times. No self-help book, therapy, or medication will free you of the inevitable disappointments that accompany a full life. Happiness is a *relative concept* in this model, since a realistic hope is that you can be happy more often than you are now. But the goal should not be total happiness or freedom from any disappointment.

Things don't always go as planned, and so we have to learn to take frustration and disappointment in stride. This means that we have to learn to keep going even if we fall down, even if friends don't always "get us," even when our work is not completely fulfilling. Inevitable disappointment doesn't mean that our relationships are dismal. No, it means that along with the good there will be some that is not so good, that our loved ones and ourselves will be completely human and will make mistakes. It means that we need to find the *balance that matters*.

How do you respond to disappointments? When a friend lets you down do you see it as a personal betrayal, a catastrophe, or something that only happens to you? Or do you think that friendships often involve disappointments? For example, isn't it likely that we will disappoint our friends? When your work—or your boss or colleagues—don't act in ways that you would like, do you then think, "I can't believe that they did that?" Is your life often characterized by a sense that you can't believe that people do what they do?

What if you changed your view of disappointment and thought that if people did half of what you would want them to do you could be satisfied? All of us are imperfect, sometimes we are petty, sometimes we let each other down. What if you built that into your expectation about what is normal?

Just as the weather can be beautiful, stormy, inclement, or unpredictable, our lives can also be this way. It comes with the territory. This doesn't make you are a cynic. It simply means that you have to be prepared for what is likely to happen. Maybe today is a stormy day, but the weather might change.

If we can realistically expect some disappointments in life, we don't have to give up and become hopeless when they occur.

How would you think and feel if you normalized being disappointed at times—even with yourself?

_____

_____

_____

_____

_____

Constructive Discomfort

Think of something that you accomplished in your life, something you did that was important to you, such as learning a skill, graduating from a program, helping a friend or family member in need, or overcoming an obstacle that seemed almost impossible for you. How much discomfort was involved? My guess is that if you acquired a skill (like learning a language, musical instrument, or athletic ability) it required time, frustration, and discomfort. It required doing something that was hard to do. The same thing is true in overcoming anxiety, which requires tolerating the discomfort of anxiety as you pursue valued goals. If you want to overcome a fear of flying, you need to fly while you are anxious. If you want to have a meaningful intimate relationship, you will have to tolerate some discomfort, disappointment, and frustration. *It won't always be on your terms.*

You may say, "I am already uncomfortable—why do I need to have more discomfort?" That's understandable. But I am not talking about tolerating discomfort as some masochistic lifestyle. I am talking about tolerating discomfort to accomplish valued goals. This is constructive in that it acknowledges that making things better often involves uncomfortable feelings. When you talk to someone studying ballet and you ask them, "How was your workout?" they say, "Good, it hurt good." In other words, it was the right discomfort—it was discomfort that reflected the feeling of pushing themselves harder, doing the demanding exercise. And they could feel it. It was discomfort that had a purpose—it was *constructive discomfort*.

Think about discomfort as a means to an end—you will need to tolerate discomfort to accomplish your goals. Think of discomfort as an investment in yourself: "I will tolerate discomfort to build my future." Think about discomfort as a tool: "I will use my discomfort to get what I want in life."

Are you willing to tolerate discomfort? How? What are some uncomfortable things that you would be willing to do?

_____

_____

_____

_____

How would your life be better if you could tolerate discomfort while pursuing a valued life?

_____

_____

_____

_____

Do What You Don't Want to Do

Making progress in life often involves doing things we don't want to do. Let's take the problem of losing weight. Despite all the diets and theories out there, it really comes down to consuming fewer calories and burning up more. What are you willing to do to accomplish your goals? Are you willing to do what needs to be done?

The question isn't "What do you *want* to do?" The real question is "What are you *willing* to do?" If you are honest about what you want to do, you might say that you want to eat a lot of food and lie on the couch eating junk food, drinking beer, and watching videos.

But progress means *do what you don't want to do so that you can get what you want to get.*

We often stubbornly demand that we don't want to do something. "I don't want to study." "I don't want to exercise." "I don't want to take a risk." "I don't want to do any of the work in this workbook." It's as if we think our lives will be great, fulfilling, and meaningful if we just do what we want to do. But real progress and real life means doing what you don't want to do. A better life doesn't just happen. It's a consequence of what we choose to do—or not do.

Why should you do what you don't want to do? *Because that is the way to reach your goals.* Once you discipline yourself—once you are willing to choose what needs to be done to accomplish your goals and live a valued life—and once you are in charge of yourself, then you will feel empowered.

I want you to get to the point where you say with pride, "I do the hard things."

How would you think and feel if you were more willing to do what you don't want to do?

_____

_____

_____

_____

_____

Successful Imperfection

One of the problematic beliefs that makes progress difficult is the thought that you need to be perfect to make progress. One of my patients told me years ago that an important idea in Alcoholics Anonymous is "make progress not perfection." This captures exactly the right idea that you can do better and better without doing the best each time. For example, perhaps you think that you should work out for one hour four days per week to get into shape. That would be wonderful, but right now you might be working out zero hours per week. So, we make progress imperfectly if we aim for twenty minutes of a light workout three times per week. Anything that moves you in the right direction is progress. You can gain success by doing things imperfectly that move you forward. Each step forward counts as progress. The problem with many of us is the idea that it has to be absolutely the best to count as progress.

Over the years I have worked with a number of publishers who told me that there are people who get contracts to write books but never write the book. These are often academic researchers who are brilliant, who have something important to say, but who cannot get their act together to get it done. They often procrastinate because they cannot get the exact, right thing down on paper. So nothing is ever finished. They often wait to feel inspired, to feel ready.

I said to one of my editors, "I don't understand. I thought they wanted to write a book." He replied, "They say they want to write a book, but what they mean is that they wish they *had written a book.*"

An accomplished artist told me that you have to look at painting like a job where you go to your studio every day. A successful playwright told me, "You don't make progress waiting for the muses." Working daily toward your goals, doing things imperfectly, reworking what is done, and being able to settle for more rather than the best will help you make progress. *Successful imperfection is how successful people think.*

What would you be able to do if you pursued things imperfectly?

_____

_____

_____

_____

_____

Flexible Satisfaction

We all have expectations about our relationships, work, income, physical well-being, and how we live. But then we treat these expectations as if they are necessities: "It is necessary that I have a job that is totally fulfilling" or "I expected that I would be further ahead than where I am." How stuck are you on these expectations about work, relationships, and how you live?

Some people are *maximizers* who expect things to be outstanding, excellent, and the best every time. And other people are *satisfiers* who expect that things could be good but are willing to settle for less than perfect. The research on maximizers and satisfiers shows that maximizers have difficulty making decisions, are less satisfied with the outcome, and experience greater regret. How "maximum" can it be if this style of thinking, expecting, and demanding makes you miserable?

We often treat our expectations as if they are *requirements* or *laws for living*. Someone might say, "I expected that I would be married by now" and then feel despondent and defeated that they don't have what they expected. Or they might say, "I expected I would be further along in my career at this point," only to feel more like a failure. I asked one of my clients, "Where did you get this expectation?" She looked at me as if my question was bizarre. It never occurred to her that expectations are *arbitrary*—no one is born with expectations about relationships and work. These are expectations that you might have learned from your parents or your friends, but they are totally arbitrary.

If expectations are arbitrary, then you can change your expectations at any time. One way to think about this concept is to ask how you would feel if you changed your expectation to match where you are right now. For example, Andy was out of work and he expected that within six weeks he would have another job. I asked him to consider the possibility of being more flexible about time—give himself a couple of more months. The pressure lifted from him and he could then allow himself more time.

Another way of thinking about expectations is to imagine how you could be satisfied with what you already have. We are often inundated with images of people who are wealthy, beautiful, and famous, and almost none of us will measure up to these standards. (Not that people who are wealthy, beautiful, or famous are really that happy. It's not what you have that counts, it's what you think you need—what you must have—that will make you unhappy.) But imagine if you could be satisfied with what you have right now. For example, are there people who are single, not wealthy, not famous, not beautiful, and not the life of the party—are any of those people experiencing satisfaction? What if you decided to work toward accepting some satisfaction in the present moment, right now, with what is in your life?

Being flexible about what you can be satisfied with can free you from a lot of emotional turmoil.

How would you think and feel if you were more flexible in what you were willing to accept as satisfactory?

Take-Home Points

♦   Difficult and unpleasant emotions are part of everyone's experience.

♦   Emotions warn us, tell us about our needs, and connect us with meaning.

♦   Strong emotions can lead us or mislead us.

♦   Beliefs about emotions can make it difficult for us to tolerate our feelings.

♦   Strategies for coping with our emotions can make matters better or worse.

♦   Emotional realism means that you won't have perfect happy feelings all the time.

♦   Inevitable disappointments mean that everyone is disappointed. Normalize this.

♦   Constructive discomfort means that you will make progress if you are able to tolerate discomfort.

♦   You can't just do what you want to do if you want to get what you want to get.

♦   Successful imperfection means that you can make progress acting imperfectly.

♦   Flexible satisfaction means that you need to be open to a range of possibilities to experience satisfaction.

CHAPTER 5

My Emotions Will Go on Forever

If you have ever had a panic attack, you know how frightening it can be. Your heart starts beating rapidly, you are short of breath, your body starts shaking, and you think that these intense, terrifying sensations will go on forever—and kill you or drive you crazy. Intense anxiety often carries that message of permanence, that it will never end. But in the many years of treating clients who have had panic attacks, I have never seen a client come in having a panic attack. All panic attacks come to an end. They are self-limiting. What goes up must come down.

And the same can be said about other emotions that we experience.

Let's take anger—another intense emotion that often feels overwhelming, out of control, and completely engulfs us. But if you think back to the most intense anger you have ever felt, I am willing to bet that right at this moment that anger is either a lot less or has completely disappeared. It's as if the tidal wave that consumed you has receded and now the waters seem calm.

Have you ever had any of the following thoughts about your emotions?

I will feel lonely forever.

This sadness won't go away.

I will be angry about this forever.

I will never feel happy again.

My feelings of hopelessness will last indefinitely.

I will never stop crying over this.

These are very common beliefs to have about intense emotions. We may believe that the feeling will be permanent. Let's look at how this way of thinking affects us—and adds to our sense of despair.

Why Do We Think Our Emotions Will Last Forever?

Our emotions evolved to protect us and guarantee that we pass on our genes. Our emotions did not evolve to make us happy, content, or even easy to get along with. Fears—such as the fear of heights, water, strangers, and closed spaces—evolved because those situations could kill us. You could fall off a cliff, drown in the lake, be killed by a stranger, or trapped in a closed space by a predator. *Fears protect.*

Sadness teaches us that we should give up on a lost cause, that pursuing something in the way that we are pursuing it is not worth it and that we should find an alternative.

For these emotions to give us a convincing message they have to scare us. They have to motivate us to do something—such as escape, avoid, attack, or try harder. Emotions have to be alarming enough, disturbing enough, and loud enough to get us to pay attention. So what better way than to hear the clear, cogent, convincing, and catastrophic message from the voice in our head:

This will last forever!

Something terrible is happening!

And attached to that alarm is another blasting message:

Unless you do something!

It has to be something that you pay attention to. Evolution cannot rely on subtlety or ambiguity. It has to send a clear, cogent, convincing, and catastrophic message. The message might be, "You will die if you don't get out of here," "Your anger will last forever unless you defeat them," "This feeling of contamination will last forever unless you wash it off."

On the other hand, let's imagine that your brain had evolved to be very cool, rational, reasonable, and calm about everything. Imagine if our ancestors had been Zen Homo sapiens, traversing the savannah, watching lions from a distance. So calm, so serene. Imagine if any time that a danger alarm sounded they just chilled out, took a step back into their mental turtle shell, and contemplated that "this too will pass." Imagine that they never treated an alarm as scary. Now, they might have been calm, they might not have had cold sweats and indigestion. But they might also have gotten eaten by the lion, killed by the strangers, or drowned in the lake.

"Better safe than sorry" is a better strategy when your life is at stake. The only downside of the intense fear, sadness, and anger might be the everyday misery that was the cost of survival. After all, you can be miserable, anxious, and neurotic and still reproduce and raise some neurotic kids. You can be "neurotic" but survive. Being happy does not guarantee survival, but being afraid might.

The software in our brains has a false-alarm bias that says that these feelings, sensations, thoughts, and emotions will last a very long time *unless you take action immediately.* Our emotions are really like bubbles in a carbonated beverage that eventually goes flat. But that's not how we experience them. We think our emotions will last indefinitely. But they don't.

Are We Good at Predicting Our Emotions?

Psychologists have become interested in how we predict our emotions. It's called *affect forecasting*, which is a fancy way of saying "predicting your emotions." For example, if you ask people, "How long do you think you will feel happy if you win the lottery, get married, get promoted, or get that new house you always wanted?" they typically predict that their positive emotions will last a very long time. The same thing is true when we ask people, "How long do you think you will be unhappy if you lose your job, get divorced, have a serious financial setback, or even lose a limb?" People answer, "A very long time." Most people believe that our emotions are *durable*—that is, once an intense emotion is activated, we believe it is here to stay.

But research shows the opposite is true. When something that we think is positive occurs, we tend to feel good for a while, but then our positive feelings eventually revert back to where they were before the event (Gilbert 1998; Wilson and Gilbert 2003). For example, let's say you buy your first house, which is larger than the apartment you had, and you feel excited. But after a year or so, you have gotten used to the house, you take it for granted, and it no longer seems that exciting. In addition, you now have mortgage payments, upkeep, and taxes to pay that detract from your enjoyment. We get used to the good and the bad. Even people who win the lottery eventually revert to their previous level of happiness. And people who think that a geographic solution to their problem—moving from freezing Minnesota to sunny California, for instance—eventually revert to how they felt when they lived in Minnesota (Lyubomirsky 2011).

Likewise, when something negative happens, we feel bad for a while but then revert back to where we were before the event. For example, if you get divorced you may feel lonely, sad, and resentful for a while, and think about how your life has changed for the worse. But after a period of time these negative feelings change. You no longer are having arguments with your ex-spouse, you no longer are worried about the process of divorce, and you may have found satisfaction in your friendships or a new intimate relationship.

Rather than having *durable* feelings, our feelings are usually *temporary*. We tend to go through and get through experiences, and our intense emotions dissipate with time. But it doesn't seem that way when we are feeling anxious, sad, or lonely.

What Happens When I Think My Emotions Will Last Forever?

The belief in the durability or permanence of emotion has a significant effect on how you feel, think, and act. Our research shows that this one belief is the best predictor of depression. In other words, if you think your negative feelings will last indefinitely, then you are likely to become depressed and anxious (Leahy, Tirch, and Melwani 2012).

But what if you treated your current emotion as temporary? If you do not believe in the durability of your negative emotions, you might pursue adaptive behavior. For example, you might pursue positive actions, such as contacting friends, exercising, volunteering, or challenging your thoughts. Some of us believe that our abilities are fixed—just as some of us believe our emotions are fixed and unchangeable. Stanford psychologist Carol Dweck describes this view of "ability" as fixed vs. the growth idea that abilities can change and improve (Dweck 2006). Similarly, you may believe that your ability to have a positive emotion can grow, change, and is within your control. These beliefs about emotion lead to other emotions—either hope (growth) or helplessness (fixed).

Do you think your emotions are fixed, or do you think they can change? Give some examples of when you thought an emotion would last a long time.

_____

_____

_____

_____

_____

What is the consequence for you when you think your current negative emotion will last indefinitely? What do you think, feel, and do?

_____

_____

_____

_____

_____

When we believe that our uncomfortable feelings will last forever, we tend to want to avoid that feeling in the first place. Roger, a client who had been struggling with obsessive-compulsive disorder, had a morbid fear of contamination from touching objects in his apartment. Even though he could understand that his fear of contamination was irrational, that it was extremely unlikely that he would get deathly ill, he still avoided touching these objects because he feared his anxiety about getting sick would last indefinitely. I asked Roger to predict exactly what would happen if he touched the objects. He predicted that doing the exposure work (touching these objects) would lead to an escalation of anxiety so crippling that he would not be able to work for several days. I asked Roger if he had had to miss work before when he tried exposure in the past. He said, "I have never tried exposure."

What does exposure look like? It simply means testing out the behavior you have been avoiding. For example, have you ever had the experience of standing on a beach and being too afraid of the cold water to run in? You see fifty people—many of them children—splashing around. It's 90 degrees outside and a cool swim in the ocean would feel great, but you are worried that if you get in it will be incredibly cold and that you will be freezing for the entire time that you are in the water. You finally decide, "Okay, I will give it a try." The first few minutes you feel the chill, but as you swim around and jump in the waves, you start to feel more comfortable. This is the exposure—testing the waters (pun intended!) of your fear. As it turns out, the duration of the discomfort was short—but the feeling of enjoyment lasts a lot longer.

Look at the worksheet "What I Avoid Because I Think My Emotions Will Go on Indefinitely" and list some of the behaviors and situations that you have avoided. For example, you might avoid exercise because you believe that the discomfort will last too long, or you might avoid seeing friends because you believe your anxiety will last for the entire time you are with them.

In the second column, list the negative thoughts and feelings that you have as a result of your avoidance. These might include thoughts that you are helpless, that you can't get anything done, or that you are different from everyone else. You might list feelings of defeat, hopelessness, sadness, or anger toward yourself. In the third column, list examples of events or behaviors that you did not avoid (although you were anxious) and what actually happened. Did your negative feelings last indefinitely?

What I Avoid Because I Think My Emotions Will Go on Indefinitely

Behaviors and Situations I Avoid	Negative Thoughts and Feelings I Have as a Result of Avoidance	Behaviors and Situations I Did Not Avoid— And What Happened

Will My Emotions Change?

I once had a client whose daughter had severe highs and lows. The mom was upset that her daughter was upset. I indicated that I could see that she had a great deal of empathy, compassion, and concern for her daughter, but I also asked if she could imagine that her daughter might feel some positive emotions later today or tomorrow. She smiled and said, "Yes, I have seen this happen so many times. She is crying, and then later that night I talk to her and she tells me that she had a good time with her friend." The daughter's intense negative emotions were fluid—changing from hour to hour.

We can find out if that is true for you. During the next week, I invite you to notice which of your emotions change and which remain the same. Use the worksheet "How My Emotions Change" to keep track of the negative emotions that concern you, along with their level of intensity, every hour of the week. But before you do that, take a moment to predict what you think you might discover about your emotions.

What do you think you will find if you keep track of your emotions for a week? Will you just see negative emotions every hour? Or will you find a range of positive, neutral, and negative emotions?

_____

_____

_____

_____

_____

_____

Let's take a look at how Judy filled out the worksheet. Judy, who was upset about a breakup with Mark, kept track of her emotions for an entire week. She had been worried that her loneliness, sadness, and hopelessness would persist at great intensity. But she found that her loneliness was reduced to 0 when she was talking with a friend and that her sadness was reduced to 3 when she went to a museum. She kept track of positive feelings and found that she had feelings of curiosity, closeness with friends, and appreciation of the beautiful art. She noticed that her feelings of hopelessness were less after she worked out at the gym. When she was at work, the negative emotions of loneliness, sadness, and hopelessness were a lot less. Her sadness was not fixed, it changed over the course of a few hours—every day. Not only was Judy especially bad at predicting her emotions, she was biased toward predicting only negative emotions.

Might you be like Judy? If your emotions change with time, situations, and activities, then your sense of permanence may be off. Let's find out by tracking your emotions. Select one or more emotions you want to focus on. For example, if your major concern is feeling sad, write "sadness" at the top of the table. Then rate the current intensity level of that emotion from 0 to 10, whereby 0 is none and 10 is overwhelming. Then keep track of that emotion and its intensity from 0 to 10 every hour of the week. When it is high (7 or above), write what you are doing in the second table. If you have a positive emotion that is 5 or above, list that in the table as well. For example, if you feel "interested" in something at a level of 5 at 3 p.m. Monday, write "interested 5."

I recommend that you track more than one emotion by either making a copy of the worksheet or downloading it from http://www.newharbinger.com/44802. When you are able to see that your overwhelming emotions eventually subside, you are able to have less fear and anxiety—and make more helpful choices. Let's see if the intensity of your emotions changes over the course of a day or week.

How My Emotions Change

Emotions I am concerned about: _____ Rating _____

	Mon	Tues	Wed	Thurs	Fri	Sat	Sun
7–9 a.m.							
9–11 a.m.							
11 a.m.–1 p.m.							
1–3 p.m.							
3–5 p.m.							
5–7 p.m.							
7–9 p.m.							
9–11 p.m.							
11 p.m.–1 a.m.							
1–3 a.m.							
3–7 a.m.							

	Negative Emotions (7 or Higher) and What I Was Doing	Positive Emotions (5 or Higher) and What I Was Doing
Monday		
Tuesday		
Wednesday		
Thursday		
Friday		
Saturday		
Sunday		

When you look at how your emotions change, do you notice any pattern? Are you feeling worse when you are alone or with people? Do you feel worse when you are ruminating and dwelling on your feelings, or when you isolate yourself and become passive? Do you feel better when you engage in behavior that gets you up and active? Or when you are engaged in productive work?

Listening to Your Past and Future Selves

If you are going through a rough time in the present moment—maybe feeling lonely, rejected, or sad—you may believe that this is the only self that there is: the *Present Self.* But the reality is that you are an entire string of different selves across time.

Let's assume for a moment that you are twenty-eight years old. Now, let's get into a time machine that goes back to you at the ages of five, ten, fifteen, twenty, twenty-five, and last year. What were the range of feelings—positive and negative—that you had at those different ages? What were you doing when you had those positive emotions? What interested you? What turned you off? Now, as you travel back to those different selves of past years, did any emotion really remain permanent? Was there flexibility in how you experienced your life?

On the following worksheet, recall your positives memories. Go back one, five, and ten years, and back to your childhood. In the middle column, describe the positive emotions and experiences that your past selves experienced. In the third column, describe what was going on in your life, what you were feeling, and what you were thinking.

Listening to My Past Selves

Past Selves	Positive Experiences and Emotions of Past Selves	What I Thought and Felt
One year ago		
Five years ago		
Ten years ago		
As a child		

How does it feel now to think about the range of selves and experiences that you had over the course of your life?

_____

_____

_____

_____

Now, get back into the time machine. I want you to imagine yourself five, ten, twenty, and thirty years from now. These *Future Selves* are looking back to your present moment and talking to you. Think about what you want that Future Self to look like, sound like. Let's imagine that your Future Self is also your *Wise Self*. (It's possible that your Future Self could also be an impulsive self.) This Wise Self can consider all the ups and downs of your life. The Wise Self knows what is best for you in the long run. It is more rational, more in tune with your values, more in control.

When Judy imagined her Future Wise Self five years from now, she said, "Don't get too hung up on the breakup with Mark. He wasn't right for you, he wasn't able to understand and accept you. Whatever feelings you have about him, from where I am in the future you won't even think about him. We need to build a stronger Judy who doesn't need him to feel good about herself. You can start that today."

Now it's your turn. Think ahead to your Future Selves one, five, and ten years from now. Try to focus on some positive possibilities for your Future Selves. Imagine your Future Selves feeling calm, content, connected, and caring toward you. In the middle column, describe some of the positive experiences and emotions that your Future Selves might experience. In the third column, describe what might be going on in your life, what you might feel, and what you might think. How might your Future Selves advise you about your current feelings and thoughts? Can you imagine the soothing, calming, and compassionate messages that your Future Selves might share with you? Write them down.

Listening to Your Future Selves

Future Selves	Positive Experiences and Emotions of Future Selves	What Would I Think and Feel
One year from now		
Five years from now		
Ten years from now		
Twenty years from now		

How does it feel now to think about the range of selves and experiences that you might have over the course of your future life?

_____

_____

_____

_____

Our Future Self might experience a wide range of positive, neutral, or negative emotions. We don't really know what those experiences will be. But we do know that our Future Self will have some range of emotions and that whatever you feel right now might change.

What Might Help You Cope in the Future?

One reason that we believe in the durability of our emotions is that we tend to focus on how we feel right now. This is called *anchoring*. It's as if our anxiety or sadness is an anchor that drags us to the bottom and keeps us from imagining moving forward in a different direction. For example, let's imagine that you are feeling deeply sad at the present moment. Maybe you have been feeling sad most of the time for the past two days. Right now your sadness feels unbearable. You begin to think about the next month, the next year, the rest of your life. And now you think, "I will live a life of loneliness and sadness."

In the next exercise you will investigate how long your emotions actually last. Make a copy of this worksheet (or print one from http://www.newharbinger.com/44802) so that you can test it out several times during the coming week. In the first column, rate the intensity of any emotion that you're feeling right now from 0 to 10, whereby 0 is none and 10 is overwhelming. In the middle column, write down how long you think this intensity will last at this level—this is your *prediction*. For example, you might answer thirty minutes, a few hours, a day, a week, or forever. In the third column, revisit this worksheet a day or week later and indicate how long the level of intensity actually lasted.

How Long Will This Feeling Last?

Current Unpleasant Emotion and Intensity Level (0–10)	Date and Time of Emotion	How Long Do I Think It Will Last?	Actual Outcome
Anger			
Anxiety			
Sadness			
Helplessness			
Hopelessness			
Loneliness			
Other:			
Other:			
Other:			

When Judy filled out this worksheet, she was focusing on a recent breakup with Mark. She had a range of negative emotions: anger (8), anxiety (8), sadness (9), helplessness (8), hopelessness (9), loneliness (9), and desperation (9). She predicted that her feelings of despair and loneliness would last for months—maybe for a few years. There seemed no way out. But when she kept track of her actual feelings over the next week she realized that every one of those feelings changed to become less intense.

We often forget that our past negative emotions feel intense initially but eventually evaporate over time. For instance, I felt quite angry about something a colleague did a number of years ago. My anger was a 9. I took things very personally, labeled him negatively, and couldn't imagine not having angry feelings toward him. Yet, in retrospect, those feelings at the intense level lasted 30 to 60 minutes at a time, until I moved on to other things unrelated to him. My feelings further decreased in time as I realized that this wasn't a personal thing, that there were other positive goals for me, and that his behavior was irrelevant to my current and future happiness. The point is that my intense feelings changed.

In the next exercise, "What Happened to My Emotions in the Past?," describe some situations that led you to have intense negative emotions. In the second column, list the emotions that were very intense and rate them from 0 to 10, whereby 0 is none and 10 is overwhelming. These emotions might include the same emotions as in the previous exercise. In the third column, describe how long those emotions lasted at that intensity level. In the fourth column, describe the reasons why those emotions changed.

What Happened to My Emotions in the Past?

Situation I Experienced	Past Unpleasant Emotions and Intensity Level (0–10)	How Long Did They Last?	Why Did My Emotions Change?

What do you conclude about your past intense emotions?

_____

_____

_____

_____

Take-Home Points

- When you think your emotions will go on indefinitely, you feel helpless, hopeless, depressed, and more anxious.

- Your belief in the permanence of emotions leads you to avoid experiences that could help you cope better.

- We tend to overpredict how intense and permanent our emotions will be.

- Evolution built in this tendency to overpredict in order to help us escape from danger. But we are no longer facing the dangers our ancestors faced.

- Get into a time machine and go to the past and the future to notice how your emotions change.

- Think back to your emotions in the past and why they changed.

- Think ahead to your Future Self. What advice would that self give you now about the way you feel?

- What might help you cope better in the future?

CHAPTER 6

I Feel Guilty About My Feelings

Even though we all have a lot of difficult emotions, we may believe that we *shouldn't feel* the way we do. We may feel guilty about our sexual fantasies, ashamed about feeling envious of someone doing better than we are doing, guilty about our anger toward our parents and friends, or ashamed that we are feeling sad when we think we don't have a right to be depressed. These feelings of shame and guilt add a heavy burden to the emotions that we already have.

For example, Simon told me about a man he went to college with who was doing much better than Simon was doing in his career.

"I know I shouldn't feel this way," Simon confessed, "but I really can't stand it when I hear about Ken's success. I just heard last week that Ken is getting a divorce, and I have to admit I felt good about it. I just don't like the fact that he has been happier and more successful than I have been."

Simon admitted that he felt envious of Ken, but he also felt guilty about his envy. I asked him, "Why do you feel guilty about your envy?" Simon looked at me as if I were from another planet. "You're not supposed to feel good about someone else having a problem. You shouldn't be envious of other people. It's not a nice thing to feel."

Along with feelings of guilt—whereby we think we are violating our own standards of what we should feel and think—we also have feelings of shame about our feelings. We feel shame when we think that others would think less of us. For example, people often feel ashamed about their sexual fantasies. Eduardo was having an intimate relationship with Caroline and he enjoyed sex with her. They could communicate well, they enjoyed the different ethnic restaurants in their neighborhood, and they would stay up late talking about just about anything. Caroline told Eduardo about some of her past sexual experiences with other men, and Eduardo noticed that he was getting aroused. He found both Caroline and the man he imagined exciting, and then began to fantasize about having sex with the man while he was having sex with Caroline. Eduardo always thought of himself as heterosexual and so he began to worry about his fantasies. He felt ashamed of these feelings and dreaded that Caroline might find out.

Family Myths About Emotions: You Shouldn't Feel That Way!

Many of our guilty and shameful thoughts about emotions were learned when we were growing up. Think back to when you were a kid. Which emotions were you told were not okay? Was it not okay to feel angry? Were you taught that anxiety and sadness were signs of weakness? Were you humiliated when you cried? Did you learn that certain sexual desires and fantasies were bad? Were you taught that having certain emotions and expressing them—for example, crying—was childish, weak, annoying, or manipulative? What were the "emotion messages" that you learned from your parents, teachers, siblings, and friends?

Keith's Story

Another client of mine was Keith, who played professional football until his career ended rather abruptly when he suddenly—for no apparent reason—could not stand, walk, or run very well. No injury was revealed on examination. Keith was a large man, physically well-built, but he had a quiet demeanor, speaking in a soft voice. He was a devout Christian who prayed daily and lived with his mother, who was a very controlling and critical person. They would sit at home in her apartment and watch television shows that had "good values."

As he was talking with me he said, "I think it is better for me to lie on the floor because I feel more comfortable that way." He then stretched himself on the floor in my office and continued to talk about his desire to get rid of all of his anger. "My anger is bad—it's dirty anger." Keith believed that thoughts and feelings of anger and resentment were bad and that he needed to eliminate them completely. As he was lying on the floor one day, he described how he resented his mother's nagging. He clearly felt angry at her, but he would say, "I know she is trying to be helpful."

I encouraged Keith to talk more about his anger. As he did, he began rising from the floor, and I could see the physical strength in his arms and shoulders. His voice become louder—not too loud—but no longer the whisper that was sometimes barely audible. I said, "I notice as you talk about your anger toward your mother that you seem physically stronger and you began sitting up. Why is that?" He then quickly lay down and I asked him why he was lying on the floor again. "I am afraid of my anger. I shouldn't feel this way. It's dirty anger."

The emotion messages we received as children from adults may also have included labeling messages—we were labeled by the emotions we showed. Do any of the following seem familiar?

- ☐ If you cry, you are weak.
- ☐ If you are afraid, you are a coward.
- ☐ If you are sad, you are selfish,
- ☐ You shouldn't feel upset, because you have things better than other kids do.
- ☐ You are making me upset with your crying.
- ☐ Other kids are able to handle things, why can't you?
- ☐ Get over it.
- ☐ Grow up.
- ☐ Stop bothering me with this.
- ☐ Can't you see I have my own problems?
- ☐ You don't make any sense.
- ☐ You just go on and on.
- ☐ I can't stand listening to you.

Sometimes parents and friends think that they are supportive when they say the following:

Don't worry, everything will work out.

You will get over it.

It's not a big deal.

Get your mind off of it.

Other people have it worse.

The problem with these "supportive" comments is that they invalidate you and sound dismissive of your feelings. They may make you believe that your emotions are not important to other people—that you should just start feeling better because people tell you it's okay. Although parents and friends may be well-intentioned, it's important for you to feel that others not only care about your feelings but have the time and interest in letting you share those feelings.

Which messages made you feel ashamed or guilty about your feelings?

_____

_____

_____

Which messages made you feel that others had little interest in your feelings?

_____

_____

_____

Which "supportive" messages from parents or friends are the least helpful when you are upset?

_____

_____

_____

Which emotions or desires do you feel ashamed or guilty about?

_____

_____

_____

Wanda's Story

Wanda was someone who could tolerate some emotions just fine but not others. She had a good job, a young child, and a loving husband, but she felt guilty that she was sad and depressed. When she came to see me, I asked her, "Why do you feel guilty about your depression?"

"Because I have everything that I should want," Wanda replied. "Other people are worse off than I am, but I am depressed. I wonder if I am just selfish."

"You are thinking that depression is a choice and that somehow you are a selfish person for feeling sad."

"Yeah, I guess I do."

I mentioned to Wanda that there could be a number of reasons for her depression. She shared that her father drank a lot and that he was probably depressed. And that he didn't like to talk about his feelings. Her mother was always worried, but she would try to keep it to herself. One of her uncles had been hospitalized with depression. With both of her parents having difficulties, and perhaps some psychological problems running in the family, I questioned whether part of her depression could be genetic.

"I guess that is possible," said Wanda. "Yeah. But I have all these other good things in my life."

"You said that in your family people didn't talk about negative feelings."

"Well, the idea was that we had a good life—that is, we had money—and you were supposed to show everyone how good things are. We had to look good."

"So there was no place for sadness, anxiety, or loneliness?"

"You were supposed to keep those feelings to yourself."

"Do you think that you learned to be ashamed or guilty about these emotions?"

"Come to think of it, that is exactly what happened."

"And now it is happening again. You are making yourself guilty about your depression. It is hard enough to be depressed, but even more difficult to feel depressed about being depressed."

Wanda felt guilty about her sadness because she thought that she had a good life and did not have a right to her sadness. She also had feelings of shame because she thought others would think that she was spoiled and did not appreciate what she had. These guilty and shameful feelings added to her sadness and sense of being undeserving—they made her more depressed.

We can fear that others will judge us for our feelings, and we can also believe that our feelings are morally wrong. Given this way of thinking, consider how your feelings, fantasies, or desires have been impacted. For example, let's say you feel envious that someone is doing better than you have been doing. Maybe you think that their advantage is unfair. Your envy involves other emotions—such as anxiety, sadness, and even anger. Okay. So you have all of these difficult emotions. But then you have another set of thoughts about your envy: "Only a petty and mean person is envious" and "If people knew I was envious they would think less of me." So now you feel guilty and ashamed about your envy, and this makes you more anxious and depressed.

Take a look at the diagram "Thoughts and Feelings About Envy." It illustrates how you can have a difficult emotion—envy—and then have negative thoughts about yourself for having this emotion. These are your *emotions about an emotion*—and, in this case, it makes it hard for you to tolerate the feelings that you have.

Thoughts and Feelings About Envy

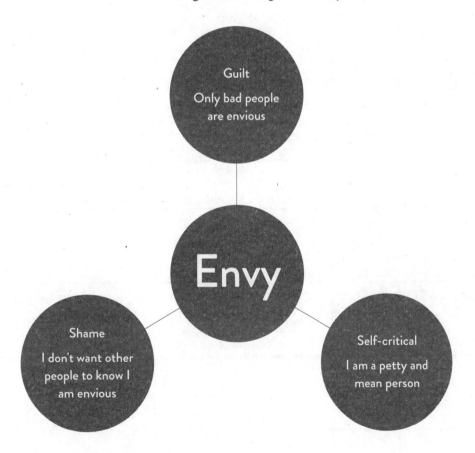

We have a lot of emotions that we find unpleasant at times. In the exercise that follows, indicate whether any of the listed emotions cause you to feel guilty or ashamed for having them. Then, in the third column, indicate why you feel guilty or ashamed.

Emotions I Feel Guilty or Ashamed About

Emotion	Yes/No	Why I Feel Guilty or Ashamed
Anger		
Sadness		
Anxiety		
Fear (phobia)		
Loneliness		
Helplessness		
Hopelessness		
Jealousy		
Envy		

Emotion	Yes/No	Why I Feel Guilty or Ashamed
Boredom		
Lack of interest		
Sexual desire		
Stress		
Frustration		
Confusion		
Ambivalence		
Other:		
Other:		
Other:		

Why Shouldn't You Have the Feelings That You Have?

We often think that there are good emotions and bad emotions. For example, some people think that happiness is a good emotion and that jealousy is a bad emotion. It's as if an emotion is a moral failing: "I am jealous, that's a bad emotion, therefore I am bad." But we wouldn't think the same thing about asthma: "I have asthma, asthma is a bad thing to have, therefore I am bad."

We may also confuse having an emotion with the problematic behaviors that sometimes follow from the emotion. For example, Linda thought that jealousy was a bad emotion, and she then equated the feeling of jealousy with the idea that she would then start to berate and attack her boyfriend. But she never berated her boyfriend.

Having a feeling (for example, anger) is not the same as acting on it (for example, being hostile). We hold people responsible for their actions—for example, their hostile behavior—but not for their internal emotions. In fact, making a choice—indeed, making a moral choice—would involve recognizing that you have a desire to take an action, *but you choose not to*. For example, you may recognize that you have a desire to attack someone verbally (a behavior) but you choose not to take that action. You resisted the urge to act.

What Are the Consequences of Your Guilt and Shame About Your Emotion?

You feel worse. And the reason you feel worse is that you have added guilt and shame to envy, which already involves anxiety, sadness, and anger. As you criticize yourself for your emotion, you begin to focus your attention on it—"I am feeling envious again"—and then you dwell or ruminate on your emotion—"What is wrong with me that I feel this way?" As you feel ashamed about your emotion, you will hide these feelings from other people. This leads you to think, "I must be the only person who feels this way." This adds to your sense of humiliation, shame, and guilt, and you begin wondering even more, "Why do I have these feelings?"

As you harbor these envious feelings and dwell on them, you become more depressed and more doubtful about your right to these feelings. Then you begin thinking that no one could possibly understand you since you are so different from everyone else. You may say to yourself, "These are *bad* feelings," and then you start watching your feelings to see if you have more bad feelings. You begin to get hyperfocused on your bad feelings, and then you conclude that you are completely filled with these feelings and that there is little else about you except these feelings.

Think about some of the emotions that you have had in the past: anger, resentment, envy, jealousy, hopelessness. Are there times when you did not act on these emotions? Why didn't you act on those emotions?

_____

_____

_____

_____

_____

_____

Is there some moral rule that says you shouldn't have these feelings? What is the rule and where did it come from?

_____

_____

_____

_____

Having an emotion is not a choice—it is an experience. It's like indigestion. How can having an experience be immoral?

_____

_____

_____

_____

What if you thought of emotions as simply a mental event rather than an immoral choice? What if an emotion is simply a biochemical event in your brain? Would you feel less ashamed and guilty?

_____

_____

_____

_____

Now let's try another exercise. Think about an emotion that bothers you—one that you feel either guilty or ashamed about. List that emotion in the left column. Then in the middle column, circle the behavior that you engage in when you feel guilty or ashamed about this emotion. In the right column, list some examples of those behaviors. To practice this exercise with other emotions, make a copy of this worksheet or download it from this book's website at http://www.newharbinger.com/44802.

The Consequences of My Guilt or Shame

Emotion	What I Think or Do	Examples
	Criticize myself	_____ _____ _____ _____
	Blame other people	_____ _____

Emotion	What I Think or Do	Examples
	Hide my feelings from people	_____
		_____
	Isolate myself from people	_____
	Decrease any positive activity	_____
		_____
	Ruminate and dwell on my feelings	_____
	Worry about the future	_____
		_____
	Binge eat	_____
	Drink alcohol	_____
	Use drugs	_____
	Try to distract myself	_____
	Ask people for reassurance	_____
	Complain to other people	_____
	Other behavior:	_____
		_____

What do you think about the consequences of your feeling guilty and ashamed? Do they add to your unhappiness? Answer the following questions to explore more on this topic.

When you feel ashamed or guilty do you start focusing more on those bad feelings? How does focusing on bad feelings affect you?

_____

_____

_____

_____

_____

_____

Are you less likely to share your feelings with other people? Why? _____

_____

_____

_____

_____

If you don't share those feelings, do you then think you are completely different from other people? ___

_____

_____

_____

_____

Do you dwell on why you have these feelings and then feel worse?

_____

_____

_____

_____

_____

_____

Why do you think your emotions are not legitimate?

_____

_____

_____

_____

_____

_____

You can feel ashamed or guilty about a wide range of feelings, fantasies, and desires. Some people feel ashamed about their sexual fantasies. Others feel guilty that they have desires for revenge. Many of my clients believe that they don't have a right to feel a certain way. I ask them, "Do people have a right to have asthma? If depression is an illness like asthma, don't you have a right to have an illness?"

We can even ask what it means to say that an emotion is not legitimate. For example, we don't say that asthma, high blood pressure, or indigestion are illegitimate. We don't say, "You don't have a right to your indigestion." That's because we don't think of physical ailments as moral issues. We think of them as physical experiences. What if we thought of an emotion as a physical experience with a sense of awareness of that experience: "I am having feelings of anger that I notice right now."

Does it really make sense to question whether an emotion is legitimate? Why or why not?

_____

_____

_____

_____

Would you think that a headache was not legitimate? Why?

_____

_____

_____

_____

Are there some good reasons why you might feel the way you feel? What are they?

_____

_____

_____

_____

What if you accepted your unpleasant emotion as an experience rather than judge yourself for having it? What would be different for you?

_____

_____

_____

_____

Why Do You Judge Your Emotions?

There are so many things about ourselves that we do not judge—or at least that we shouldn't judge. For example, we generally don't judge someone because they are left-handed or three inches taller or have brown eyes. Why do we need to judge our emotions?

Think about how liberating it will be for you if you let go of judging your emotions and simply *observe and accept* the emotions that you have. Rather than think, "I must be a bad person because I envy my friend's success," you can instead think, "Oh, I can see that I am having an envious feeling right now. That is a feeling I have sometimes." And you might go even further: "Almost everyone has feelings of envy at times."

Perhaps you think that if you don't judge your feeling you will lose control. Your theory is that you have to criticize yourself for your feelings or else you will take action that will be morally wrong or harmful in some way. But this may not be true.

For example, let's imagine that you are negotiating with your boss about a raise. You notice that you are feeling angry with your boss because she seems to be stubborn. You notice the anger, but rather than judge the anger as bad or judge yourself as bad, you simply acknowledge to yourself that you have that feeling right now. When you acknowledge that feeling you accept it right now as a "given." You might say to yourself, "I notice that I am angry, and I need to remind myself that I need to relate to my boss in a professional way." You recognize that it is okay to feel angry—and that it might be the way other people feel—but you are not going to let that guide your actions. You can accept the feeling of anger right now without acting in a hostile way.

Or perhaps you think that if you don't judge your emotion and judge yourself, then you are giving yourself permission to be irresponsible. After all, you wouldn't say to yourself, "It's okay to steal" or "It's okay to punch someone." But being nonjudgmental about an emotion is not saying it is okay to act in an irresponsible way. It is simply being honest about the way you feel. Noticing, observing, labeling, and being aware of your emotion may actually help you have better control, so that you don't harm other people or yourself with your actions.

For this next exercise, think about emotions you have that you judge yourself for having. Write these down in the left column. In the middle column, circle the reasons for feeling guilty or ashamed about your feelings. In the right column, write out your explanation for how this makes sense today. For example, if you say that anger is a bad emotion that you should never have because this is how you were brought up, indicate in the right column how this makes sense or does not make sense now that you are an adult. We often have a different view of things as we mature and go through different experiences.

Why I Need to Judge My Emotions

Emotions I Judge Negatively	Reasons for Judging My Emotions	Explanation of How This Makes Sense or Doesn't Make Sense Today
	Religious reasons.	
	This is how I was brought up.	
	This is how other people judge these emotions.	
	To make sure I do the right thing.	
	I have no choice.	
	I have a responsibility to judge these feelings.	
	Only bad or weak people have these feelings.	
	Other:	
	Other:	
	Other:	

If you notice an emotion without judging yourself, will you really lose control of your actions? Why or why not?

_____

_____

_____

_____

_____

Being honest about the way you feel may be the first step in avoiding problematic behavior. Can acknowledging a feeling and accepting it help you choose not to act on the feeling?

_____

_____

_____

_____

If everyone has emotions like this, maybe this makes you human, not bad. What if you thought of these emotions as part of being a human being? How would you feel then?

_____

_____

_____

_____

If Someone Else Had This Feeling, Would You Think Less of Them?

We are often more understanding about other people than we are about ourselves. For example, Linda could understand that it was okay for her friends to have jealous feelings, but she was critical of herself for having these feelings: "I can understand why my friend Diane feels jealous because her boyfriend flirts a lot—but I don't think he means anything by it. But I feel that my jealousy is out of control. I just feel so anxious when I get jealous."

What Linda is concerned about is her feeling of anxiety—but she can accept that other people have the same feelings. She has a *double standard*. We often think that we should hold ourselves to a higher standard than we apply to other people. This is clearly unfair to us and only adds to our guilt and shame.

As another example, Wanda told me that one of her friends, Sandy, had given up her work as a lawyer in order to raise her children and be supportive to her husband and his ambitious career. She told me that she understood why her friend Sandy felt sad, lonely, helpless, bored, and frustrated. In fact, Wanda was quite supportive to her friend. She told her, "You worked so hard to become a lawyer, and now you feel isolated and not fulfilled in simply being a stay-at-home mom. I understand that it feels confusing to you since you love your children and you want to be supportive to Dan. But you also have a life to live of your own. I know exactly how you feel since I have had a lot of the same feelings."

Now let's see if you can identify some of the emotions that you may have been feeling—maybe guilt or shame—and ask yourself how you would think of someone else with these feelings. On the following worksheet, try to give an example of someone you know or have known. Describe how you feel about them and what you might say to them.

How I Would Think of Someone Else with These Feelings

Emotion	Person Who Has Felt This Way, How I Feel About Them, and What I Would Say to Them
Anger	
Sadness	
Anxiety	
Fear (phobia)	
Loneliness	
Helplessness	
Hopelessness	
Jealousy	
Envy	
Boredom	
Lack of interest	

Sexual desire	
Stress	
Frustration	
Confusion	
Ambivalence	
Other:	
Other:	
Other:	

If you think it is okay for someone else to have the same feelings that you have, why do you use a different standard for yourself?

_____

_____

_____

_____

_____

_____

Accept Your Feelings: They Simply Are Your Feelings

Imagine if you eliminated your guilt and shame, and you simply accepted your emotion without any judgment of your feeling or of yourself. *It simply is.* You can accept the emotion as an experience that you have right now. You don't need to judge yourself. Helpful ways of responding to your guilt and shame include the following: you can normalize that other people have these feelings, you can recognize that having a feeling doesn't mean you act on it, and you can understand that no one is hurt by your feelings.

Sometimes we think that we need to feel guilty or ashamed about our feelings or thoughts in order to keep ourselves from acting on them. This confuses our inner experiences with our behaviors. Every day you may have a feeling or a thought about something and choose not to act on it. For example, let's say you are trying to lose weight and the dessert menu is handed to you while you're in a restaurant. You have a craving for chocolate cake, but then you think, "I might enjoy that cake but I don't need the calories," so you choose not to order it. You had a desire for the cake but you made a choice not to act on your desire. Your desires, thoughts, and feelings are different from the choice to act.

By being honest with yourself that you have a feeling, you actually can have more control over your behavior. This is very obvious when you are dieting. You need to recognize that you have the desire for the high-calorie food so that you don't simply act on impulses. You don't want to be blindsided by your desires and appetites.

When Brenda was trying to lose weight, she anticipated her desire for high-calorie foods and chose to not to have that kind of food around; she reminded herself that she didn't have to be controlled by her desires.

You might think, "Won't feeling guilty about my desires give me more control?" No—it will give you less control. For example, feeling guilty about your hunger for the cake will make you more anxious and depressed, and this will make you more likely to overeat. You will eat the cake to calm your anxiety and guilt.

Rather than feeling guilty or ashamed about your emotions, you can practice a number of techniques that we've touched on in this chapter:

- Notice the emotion.

- Label the emotion.

- Accept that the emotion is here right now.

- Realize that other people have the same feelings.

- Recognize that an emotion is not the same thing as acting on an emotion.

- Show some compassion toward yourself for having a difficult time with your feelings.

Now let's try one more exercise on this subject. On the worksheet that follows, list the emotions that you find difficult. They might include anger, jealousy, anxiety, sadness, or helplessness. Now, rather than feel guilty or ashamed about your emotion, think of how you could accept these feelings without being self-critical.

What If I Didn't Feel Guilty or Ashamed?

Emotion	Helpful Ways to Think About My Emotion

If you feel less guilt or shame about your feelings, will you be less emotional about your emotions?

_____

_____

_____

_____

_____

_____

Can you make decisions about what action to take without feeling guilty about your feelings? Describe.

_____

_____

_____

_____

_____

_____

Take-Home Points

- We learn about our emotions from our family, friends, and partners. Think about the messages and myths that you learned.

- Sometimes we learn that certain emotions are bad to have, and then we feel ashamed and guilty about our feelings.

- Feelings are not the same thing as choices. You can feel angry without acting in a hostile way.

- Feeling guilty about an emotion intensifies that emotion and makes us more anxious.

CHAPTER 7

My Emotions Are Out of Control

Yes, unpleasant and unfair things happen to us, but we often can make things worse or better depending on how we think about things. If you think that something is terrible—rather than unpleasant or inconvenient—then you are going to be more upset. If you think that everyone should like you, then you will be frustrated and feel rejected on a regular basis. If you think that the future is bleak, then you will feel hopeless. Every time you are upset about something, lurking behind your emotion are the thoughts that fuel your feelings. Thoughts are both the fuel and the map, and it is up to you to decide not to step on the accelerator and go over the cliff. You have choices.

If you are going to have more control over your emotions it might be helpful to consider alternative ways of thinking about what has happened. In each of the examples above, it may be that your feelings are a result of specific ways of thinking. But there is always another way to see things, and changing your thinking might dramatically affect how you feel.

Larry's Story

When Larry came into a session, his girlfriend, Anna, had sent him a text message that she was breaking up with him. The relationship had been up and down since the beginning, a few months ago. Although Larry told me that he felt a special connection to Anna, he also said that she was often critical, unreliable, and unaffectionate. When he got the text message saying good-bye, he felt overwhelmed with emotions.

I asked him what feelings he was having and he said, "Angry. Anxious. Confused. And sad." On closer inspection of his feelings, he also said he felt a little relieved because he was getting off the roller coaster. But as the week progressed he said he felt overwhelming anxiety. I asked him, "When you are feeling anxious it is usually about something you are thinking. Try to finish this sentence with the first thoughts that come to your mind: I am feeling anxious because I think…"

"…I will never find a partner."

"And if I never find a partner, that makes me anxious because I think…"

"…I could never be happy without someone to love."

"And the reason I think I would never find a partner is…"

"…Anna broke up with me. Maybe there is something wrong with me."

"And if there is something wrong with me then…"

"…No one would want to be with me."

Essentially, everything that Larry was saying was adding to his anxiety: that he'll never find a partner, that there is something wrong with him, and that no one would want him because there is something wrong with him. This would make anyone upset. But I reminded Larry that a thought is not the same thing as reality. For example, I shared that I can have the thought that I am a zebra, but when I check it out in the mirror I don't have stripes and I don't walk on all fours. This made Larry laugh.

Is That Alarm for Me?

Let's imagine that you are in your house and you hear an alarm—it sounds like fire trucks coming down the street. The first thought that you have is, "My house is on fire!" And then you think, "I will be burned alive!" How would you feel? Frightened, panicked? What would you do? You might check to see if there is a fire in your kitchen or run outside.

But what if instead you thought, "There might be a fire six blocks from here"? How would you feel? You might feel a little curious or even indifferent. What would you do? Maybe you would look out the window at the trucks going by or do nothing.

We can see that the same event—a loud siren—leads to two different reactions. In one, you think your house is on fire and you will be burned alive, in the other you think the fire is six blocks away and you don't have any strong emotions. When we use the *cognitive therapy* approach, we can notice what we are saying to ourselves, acknowledge how this makes us think and act, and determine if there is another way to look at things.

There is always another way to look at things. Changing your view of things can be immensely helpful. The more frequently you experiment with and practice the techniques in this chapter, the more you will see your ability to cope with emotions improve. But it takes time and practice and discipline.

Our Biased Thinking

Have you noticed that you often jump to conclusions, see things as far worse than they turn out to be, and view many things that happen in terms of the way things "should" be, rather than simply describing and accepting the world as it is? This doesn't mean that your feelings are not real, it doesn't mean that you can't be right about things being bad, and it doesn't mean that morality and rules don't count. But it might be that you have habitual patterns of thinking that escalate your emotions and make you prone to anxiety and depression.

A very powerful way of changing our feelings is to think about the situation in a different way. This is the hallmark of cognitive therapy, which was developed by Aaron Beck and Albert Ellis. It's a form of therapy that has been shown to be effective for depression, anxiety, anger, couples issues, substance abuse, and schizophrenia (Beck et al. 1979; Ellis and Harper 1975; Leahy 2018). Cognitive therapy focuses on your "cognitions," or thoughts. It proposes that our feelings are often the result of how we think about things. We call these negative thought biases *automatic thoughts* because they occur spontaneously and seem plausible. People who are depressed believe in the *negative triad*—a negative view of the self, experience, and future—with thoughts such as "I am a loser," "This is a terrible experience for me," and "The future is hopeless."

People who are prone to anxiety have their "threat detectors" operating on an ongoing basis, scanning their experience for signs of rejection, failure, or danger. Examples of this threat-detection bias include beliefs that other people don't like us, that we will fail on a task, or that our anxiety will escalate to a panic attack and we'll go insane or die. And people who are prone to anger tend to view other people as blocking them for getting what they want, humiliating them, provoking them, or insulting them (Beck 1999; DiGiuseppe and Tafrate 2007). Examples include the belief that others are in our way, that they are disrespectful, or that they are treating us with contempt. Couples in conflict tend to have one person believing that their partner should know what they want without them having to tell them, that everything should be going great at all times, and that they shouldn't have to compromise (Epstein and Baucom 2002).

If you see yourself in any of these patterns, then you are not alone. We all have biases in our thinking. It is human nature. We sometimes think ourselves into the idea that the world is a terrible place or that there is something fundamentally wrong with us. But we can examine these biases, or distortions, in our thinking and see if they really make sense.

Let's look at some common biases in thinking, starting with you. You can do this by prompting yourself: "I am upset because I am thinking…" You might answer, "… that my boss will criticize me." And then you can go further: "And if my boss criticizes me, that would make me upset because then I might get fired." And then: "If I got fired that would be upsetting because that would mean I am a failure." And finally: "If I am a failure no one will want to be with me, and then I will be alone forever, and then I could never be happy, and then life would not be worth living."

Well, maybe you don't go that far with your negative thoughts. But many people who are prone to depression and anxiety do. You can see that each thought might have a negative bias, and each negative thought can lead you to jump to more conclusions, as it did with Larry earlier in this chapter. In cognitive therapy, we identify these thoughts, categorize them, and then test them out against logic, facts, and experience.

There are a number of categories that our thoughts may fall into. Do you see yourself having any of these types of thoughts?

Categories of Biased and Distorted Thoughts

Mind reading: You believe that you know what other people are thinking without having enough evidence. For example, "She thinks I am boring."

Fortune-telling: You make predictions about the future based on little evidence. For example, "I will get fired" or "He will reject me."

Awfulizing: You believe that events will be so awful or catastrophic that they will be unbearable. For example, "It would be terrible if she rejected me" or "My anxiety will kill me."

Labeling: You view others or yourself as having global negative traits. For example, "I am a failure" or "She is evil."

Discounting positives: You ignore or discount the positive experiences or qualities in yourself, others, or in your life and treat them as unimportant. For example, "That was an easy task, so I don't count it" or "That's what your partner should do, so why give them credit for doing it?"

Negative filter: You focus almost exclusively on the negatives and seldom notice the positives. For example, "Look at all of the people who don't like me."

Overgeneralizing: You perceive a global pattern of negatives on the basis of a single incident. For example, "This generally happens to me. I seem to fail at a lot of things."

Black-and-white thinking: You view events or people in all-or-nothing terms—either all good or all bad, without shades of gray. For example, "I get rejected by everyone" or "It was a waste of time."

Shoulds: You interpret events in terms of how things should be rather than simply focusing on what is. For example, "I should do well. If I don't, then I'm a failure."

Personalizing: You view things as personally directed toward you, or you attribute a disproportionate amount of the blame for negative events to yourself, and fail to see that certain events are also caused by others. For example, "My marriage ended because I failed."

Blaming: You focus on another person as the source of your negative feelings, and you refuse to take responsibility for changing yourself. For example, "She's to blame for the way I feel now" or "My parents caused all my problems."

Unfair comparisons: You interpret events in terms of standards that are unrealistic by focusing primarily on others who do better than you and then judging yourself inferior in the comparison. For example, "She's more successful than I am" or "Others did better than I did on the test."

Regret orientation: You focus on the idea that you could have done better in the past, rather than on what you could do better now. For example, "I could have had a better job if I had tried" or "I shouldn't have said that."

What if?: You ask a series of what-if questions, and you are never satisfied with any of the answers. For example, "Yeah, but what if I get anxious?" or "What if I can't catch my breath?"

Emotional reasoning: You let your feelings guide your interpretation of reality. For example, "I feel depressed; therefore, my marriage is not working out."

Inability to disconfirm: You reject any evidence or arguments that might contradict your negative thoughts. For example, when you have the thought "I'm unlovable," you reject as irrelevant any evidence that people like you. Consequently, your thought cannot be refuted. Another example: "That's not the real issue. There are deeper problems. There are other factors."

Judgment focus: You view yourself, others, and events in terms of black-and-white white evaluations (good/ bad or superior/inferior), rather than simply describing, accepting, or understanding. You are focused on the judgments of others as well as your own judgments of yourself. For example, "I didn't perform well in college" or "If I take up tennis, I won't do well" or "Look how successful she is. I'm not successful."

Let's see how we can categorize someone's negative automatic thoughts. Let's continue with Larry, who is going through a breakup with Anna. He thinks the experience is absolutely terrible (awfulizing), he thinks it means that he completely failed in the relationship (personalizing), he believes that Anna is a terrible person (labeling), he thinks that other people will think he is loser because she broke up with him (mind reading), that he will never be happy again (fortune-telling), that all relationships are doomed (overgeneralizing), that there is nothing in his life that is positive (discounting positives), and that she should have tried harder to make things work out (shoulds).

What Are Your Biases?

All of us can have distortions or biases in our thinking—especially when we experience intense emotions. When you feel an intense emotion, it might be helpful to think about what you are saying to yourself. During the next week, take the time to notice when you are having a strong emotion—perhaps you're feeling lonely, sad, hopeless, anxious, angry, or helpless. Then write down the thoughts you're having. By monitoring and recording your thoughts you will start gaining more control over your feelings and be able to change the way you feel, rather than get hijacked by events and your interpretations of them. This doesn't mean that you are wrong or don't have a right to your feelings. But you do have a right to cope more effectively with those feelings!

Look at the list "Example Biases for Different Emotions." Then, beginning today, list your emotions and biased thoughts on the worksheet "My Biases for Different Emotions." Next, refer to the list of biased and distorted categories and try to label the type of thought you're having. Return to this worksheet over the next week or two anytime you have a strong emotion (you can also make copies of this worksheet or download one from http://www.newharbinger.com/44802). See if you can begin to catch yourself in some habits of biased thinking.

Example Biases for Different Emotions

Emotion	Typical Thoughts	Category
Anxiety	It is terrible that she said that.	Awfulizing
	My life is falling apart.	Awfulizing
	I will fail the exam.	Fortune-telling
	I can't get anything right.	Overgeneralizing and discounting positives
Sadness	I can't stand being so sad.	Awfulizing
	I will be sad forever.	Fortune-telling
	I am helpless to make things better.	Discounting positives
Loneliness	It's terrible to be alone.	Awfulizing
	I am alone because there is something wrong with me.	Personalizing and discounting positives
	People think I have nothing going for me.	Mind reading
Anger	It's awful when someone doesn't respect me.	Awfulizing
	They should always be respectful to me.	Shoulds
	He thinks he can treat me like I am inferior to him.	Mind reading
	I should get back at her for treating me this way.	Shoulds
Jealousy	It's terrible when my partner finds other people attractive.	Awfulizing
	She thinks that he is more interesting than I am.	Mind-reading
	He is not paying attention to me because he is thinking of someone else.	Personalizing and mind reading
	She is always flirting.	Overgeneralizing

My Biases for Different Emotions

Emotion	Typical Thoughts	Category

How to Put Things in Perspective

When we are intensely emotional we often see things as blown up, out of proportion, and without a reasonable perspective. This doesn't mean we shouldn't have our emotions—but the intensity, the feeling of being overwhelmed, and our tendency to act impulsively at the moment may become a problem for us. Each of the thinking biases described earlier can be addressed by using cognitive therapy techniques. These are simple techniques that you can start using right now that can help you moderate, control, and often lessen the intensity of your feelings.

Let's give it a try.

Take a look at some of the thoughts you might have when you think that something is "awful" or you think "I can't stand it." Let's take the situation of a breakup in a relationship. This is often an intensely emotional time, and you might have the full range of negative thoughts. But the intensity of your emotions doesn't mean that your thoughts are accurate. For example, let's look at the following thoughts that you might have during a breakup:

It's awful that we have broken up.

I won't be able to stand it.

I will be alone forever.

I will never be happy again.

This means I am unlovable (or a failure).

No one could ever want me again.

Let's take the first thought: "It's awful that we have broken up." We often believe that negative events are terrible, catastrophic, and unbearable. But as bad as it may feel at the moment, let's see if there is another way of making it less awful or catastrophic. If you are in conflict with a loved one, use the following worksheet to question the idea that the conflict is awful. You can also try this exercise with any negative event, such as difficulty at work, not doing well on a test, or any stressful experience; simply copy the worksheet or download it from http://www.newharbinger.com/44802 so that you can challenge your thoughts in different scenarios.

This is not to say that what is happening is meaningless or trivial—but perhaps it might not be as awful or as catastrophic as you may think it is.

Challenging the Idea That Something Is Awful

Describe the relationship conflict or negative event. For example, if it was a conflict with someone, describe the conflict. If it was a problem at work, describe exactly what happened.

_____

_____

_____

_____

_____

List all the things you can still do even if this is true. For example, can you still see friends, go to work, exercise, learn, grow, and so forth?

_____

_____

_____

_____

What did you enjoy doing before this event or experience? What were some meaningful experiences that you had that were independent of this event, situation, or experience?

_____

_____

_____

_____

Do other people survive these situations and go on to experience good things? Can you think of how they are able to do that?

_____

_____

_____

_____

_____

Are you putting too much emphasis on how you feel right now? Sometimes we judge how bad something is by how we feel right now, ignoring how our feelings might change later.

_____

_____

_____

_____

_____

What are some new opportunities that you can enjoy? Change can also involve new possibilities, new doors opening, new opportunities.

_____

_____

_____

_____

_____

Are there rewarding and meaningful activities that you can pursue this week? List some of them.

_____

_____

_____

_____

_____

Now, let's imagine that the negative event feels more final: a relationship breakup, a job loss, a college rejection, or anything else that might apply to your life. Now you think you will be forever alone, jobless, degreeless, or whatever applies. Use the following worksheet to challenge your thoughts. Feel free to try this exercise for multiple events by making a copy or downloading the worksheet from http://www.newharbinger.com/44802.

Challenging the Idea of "Forever"

Do you have other friends and family members in your life? What are your professional skills? What other schools can you apply to? Give examples.

_____

_____

_____

_____

_____

Have you been capable of making new friends and starting new relationships? Have you applied to jobs before and been hired? Have you enrolled in other schools or classes? Describe some examples.

_____

_____

_____

_____

_____

Many people go through breakups/job losses/college rejections and start new relationships/jobs/schools later. Can you think of some examples of people who have gone through this before? Give examples.

_____

_____

_____

_____

_____

You have had other relationships/jobs/classes that ended and you have met new people/applied for new work/taken other classes. Can you give some examples?

_____

_____

_____

_____

_____

Write a one-paragraph story about how you can connect with new people in your life/apply for a new job/apply to another school. What would you have to do to make this happen? What plans can you develop that can move you in this direction?

_____

_____

_____

_____

_____

When we have conflicts we might blame ourselves, label ourselves, and feel depressed and hopeless about the future because of the way we are thinking about this. Now let's challenge the idea that a breakup, job loss, school rejection, or other conflict means that you are flawed, defective, or unlovable. See if there are different ways of viewing this.

Challenging the Idea That I Am Flawed

Are you are personalizing the conflict as if it is entirely your fault? It takes two to have a breakup, for example. How did others contribute to the problem? Give examples.

_____

_____

_____

_____

_____

Conflicts don't mean people are generally unlovable or flawed—it simply means that this particular situation didn't last or that people disagree. How does this make sense for your experience?

_____

_____

_____

_____

_____

You wouldn't conclude that someone else is unlovable or flawed because they had a conflict. Why not? Give an example. Why would you have a different standard for judging someone else? Why are you so hard on yourself?

_____

_____

_____

_____

_____

Everyone has positive and negative qualities—we like and love those qualities—so saying that an entire person is unlovable or flawed makes no sense. What are some of your positive qualities pertaining to being a good partner/worker/student/human being? Give specific examples.

_____

_____

_____

_____

If someone loved you, and then you broke up, it doesn't make sense that suddenly you became unlovable. If you lost your job, it doesn't make sense that you suddenly have no skills. If you were rejected by a college, it doesn't make sense that you suddenly are dumb. How does it make sense that you and your situation are more complicated than a simple label of bad, flawed, unlovable? Give examples.

_____

_____

_____

_____

If you did make mistakes that led to the conflict, how can you learn from these mistakes and use this information in the future? How can you grow from this experience?

_____

_____

_____

_____

_____

Challenging Your Fortune-Telling

Let's take a look at your fortune-telling habits. This type of thought includes your predictions about the future, often based on inadequate information. Statements sound like the following:

I will never be happy again.

I will always be alone.

I will get rejected by them.

I will fail at that.

I will go insane.

Many of us do fortune-telling every day. It's part of human nature to fantasize about the future—in good and bad ways—and to treat our thoughts as if they are reality. But our predictions are not facts. And if we are continually predicting the most negative outcomes, then we are likely to feel anxious, sad, helpless, and hopeless.

Because the habit of fortune-telling has implications about your current and future emotions, we need to examine this type of thought to see if there might be another way of viewing the future.Reflect on some of the predictions that you are making now or have made in the past. Use the following worksheet to test out your predictions.

Challenging Your Negative Predictions

Exactly what are you predicting will happen? How confident are you that this will happen, on a percentage scale of 0 to 100? Specify as much as possible:

_____

_____

_____

_____

_____

What is the evidence that this will happen? What is the evidence that it will not happen?

Evidence in favor: _____

_____

_____

_____

_____

Evidence against: _____

_____

_____

_____

_____

Have you made negative predictions in the past that have not proven accurate? What did you predict and what actually happened?

_____

_____

_____

_____

What is the worst, best, and most likely outcome?

• Worst: _____

_____

_____

• Best: _____

_____

_____

• Most likely: _____

_____

_____

Why is the "most likely outcome" more likely than the worst outcome?

_____

_____

_____

_____

Write down a detailed description of your worst feared outcome.

_____

_____

_____

_____

_____

List all the things that would have to go wrong for this outcome to happen.

_____

_____

_____

_____

_____

List all the things that might prevent this outcome from happening.

_____

_____

_____

_____

_____

Describe in detail three positive outcomes.

_____

_____

_____

_____

_____

When you feel overwhelmed with your emotions, it may be hard to think about techniques that you can use to put things in perspective, see things differently, challenge your thoughts, and come up with new, more adaptive, more flexible, and more realistic thoughts. The ten questions on the following worksheet can help. When you are feeling overwhelmed and unsure what to do, you can orient yourself by writing down your answers. For additional blank copies, go to http://www.newharbinger.com/44802. Try this exercise at least three different times this week.

Ten Questions to Challenge and Test Your Negative Thoughts

1. **What are you thinking when you are upset?**

_____

_____

_____

_____

2. **What are the costs and benefits to you of thinking this way?**

_____

_____

_____

_____

3. How would you feel and act if you believed this thought less?

_____

_____

_____

_____

4. Which automatic thought distortions are you using? (For example, mind reading, fortune-telling, awfu-
    lizing, personalizing, etc.)

_____

_____

_____

_____

5. What advice would you give a friend?

_____

_____

_____

_____

6. What is the evidence for and against this thought?

_____

_____

_____

_____

7. What if this thought were true? What would that mean to you and what would happen next?

_____

_____

_____

_____

8. **How likely or unlikely are the events that you predict in question 7? Why?**

_____

_____

_____

_____

9. **How would you be able to cope if something negative did happen?**

_____

_____

_____

_____

10. **What would be a more realistic way of viewing things?**

_____

_____

_____

_____

Take-Home Points

- We all have biases and distortions in our thinking.

- These biases make us prone to anxiety, sadness, anger, and other difficult emotions.

- Notice what you are saying to yourself that is making you upset.

- Determine the costs and benefits to you of thinking this way.

- Ask yourself how you would feel if you believed these thoughts less.

- There is always another way to look at things.

- Ask yourself what advice you would give a friend.

- Determine whether you are jumping to conclusions.

- You can put things in perspective.

- Examine the evidence for and against your thought.

CHAPTER 8

I Can't Stand Having Mixed Feelings

Do you have a hard time having mixed feelings? Do you think you should feel only one way about someone or a situation? Do you have difficulty making decisions because you can see both the pros and cons? Ambivalence, or mixed feelings, is part of real life, and if you cannot tolerate ambivalence you will miss out on the richness of life that can also seem contradictory.

One reason you may have trouble accepting ambivalence is that you believe in "pure mind." In other words, you believe that there is some ideal state where you know for sure what is the right thing, what is the truth. You ruminate, seek reassurance, look at all the possible permutations of things while hoping for an epiphany, a sudden insight where everything will pull together. This is a myth. Reality is complex, contradictory, and always in flux, and your mind is part of that reality.

Pure mind is part of emotional perfectionism, which you learned about in chapter 4. Emotional perfectionism is the belief that we should only have certain kinds of emotional experiences—like feeling happy, content, fulfilled, not frustrated, and so forth. Pure mind is the idea that our mind should be clear, not ambivalent, not confused. But the reality is that our minds are often chaotic.

In this chapter, we will examine ambivalence, especially how to think about it. You'll come to see that life involves tradeoffs, and that certain things come with the territory. We will learn that the problem is *not* ambivalence. It's that you *think* ambivalence is the problem. Let's look at a couple of examples.

Brenda had been seeing Mike for several months, and she began to ruminate about how she felt about him. "I don't know how I feel. I mean, sometimes I like being with him, but sometimes he annoys me. Not often, but sometimes. It's like, we have this great chemistry and we really enjoy spending time together, and he is a terrific guy. But, I don't know, sometimes I get bored talking with him. He goes on about work, and to be honest I am not really that interested in his work. I just don't know how I feel. Do I like him or not?"

As a result of her ambivalence, Brenda would sometimes focus on the few times that she felt bored talking with Mike. "What's wrong with me? What's wrong with our relationship?" And then she would worry that he wasn't the "right one" for her—that maybe she should break up with him. Even though she felt more comfortable with him than anyone she had previously been involved with, she was filled with doubts. "How can I make a commitment if I have mixed feelings? Shouldn't I be sure?" What made this more difficult for Brenda is that she realized that Mike had so many great qualities. She knew he would be a wonderful partner in many ways and that he was completely devoted to her. Brenda's ambivalence about Mike bothered her.

Nicole is in a similar predicament, but her ambivalence is regarding her job. She works for a small tech company, the hours are long, the work is unpredictable, and the head of the team is sometimes unreasonable. But she loves the content of what she does, she thinks she's learning a lot, and she thinks there is a lot of growth potential. "I don't know, they tell us to *follow our dream,* and I thought this was my dream, but sometimes it's boring, sometimes it's frustrating, and I just don't know how I feel about being here." Nicole thinks that she shouldn't feel ambivalent about her work. She thinks it should be her dream. She keeps thinking that she should be in a dream job, that she should never feel bored at work, and that there is either something wrong with her or that this is not the *right job.* Nicole can't tolerate her mixed feelings about her job.

Is it Mike, the job, or a difficulty tolerating ambivalence that's the problem?

We can have mixed feelings about our relationships, our jobs, our appearance, where we live, and even about what we eat. Some of us get trapped in our ambivalence and think we have to be clear, sure, and without any doubts in order to make decisions. We are plagued with regrets and can't see things in perspective.

You may think your problem is that you *have* mixed feelings, that it is a bad thing to have doubts about anything important in your life. But if mixed feelings are part of the richness and complexity of life, what is the problem? Maybe the problem is that you *think* mixed feelings are a problem—and then you activate rumination, reassurance seeking, procrastination, and other unhelpful strategies to solve the problem. This is part of the *myth of the pure mind*, which is another part of your emotional perfectionism.

Let's find out if you cannot accept ambivalence and whether your solutions make your problems worse.

The Ambivalence Checklist

Let's see how you are with your ambivalence. Look at the statements in the middle column. Then, using the scale below, write down the number that best corresponds to the way you think about each life domain. There are no right or wrong answers.

Scale:

1 = Strongly disagree

2 = Somewhat disagree

3 = Slightly disagree

4 = Slightly agree

5 = Somewhat agree

6 = Strongly agree

Life Domain	My Beliefs	Rating (1–6)
Work	I have a hard time with my mixed feelings.	
	I often dwell on the fact that I have mixed feelings.	
	I think I should be clear about the way I feel.	
	I think that if I have mixed feelings then something is wrong.	
	It's hard to make decisions when I have mixed feelings.	

Life Domain	My Beliefs	Rating (1–6)
Romantic Relationship	I have a hard time with my mixed feelings.	
	I often dwell on the fact that I have mixed feelings.	
	I think I should be clear about the way I feel.	
	I think that if I have mixed feelings then something is wrong.	
	It's hard to make decisions when I have mixed feelings.	
Friendships	I have a hard time with my mixed feelings.	
	I often dwell on the fact that I have mixed feelings.	
	I think I should be clear about the way I feel.	
	I think that if I have mixed feelings then something is wrong.	
	It's hard to make decisions when I have mixed feelings.	
Where I Live	I have a hard time with my mixed feelings.	
	I often dwell on the fact that I have mixed feelings.	
	I think I should be clear about the way I feel.	
	I think that if I have mixed feelings then something is wrong.	
	It's hard to make decisions when I have mixed feelings.	

Look at your responses for each domain of life. Perhaps you will notice that you are more accepting of mixed feelings about some areas of life compared to others. For example, are you more accepting of mixed feelings about where you live than about a romantic relationship? If so, why is that?

_____

_____

_____

_____

_____

Do you think that your choices or involvement with an intimate partner should not involve mixed feelings? Do you think that your work should never be frustrating or boring? Why?

_____

_____

_____

_____

_____

Do your mixed feelings make it hard for you to tolerate occasional disappointment or frustration? Does your ambivalence make it hard for you to make decisions? Describe:

_____

_____

_____

_____

Think about the areas of your life where you might accept ambivalence. For example, maybe you have friends about whom you have mixed feelings—and they may have mixed feelings about you. Is that okay with you? Why is that?

_____

_____

_____

_____

Returning to Brenda and Mike momentarily, I asked Brenda why having mixed feelings about Mike was difficult for her. She looked at me with a surprised expression and said, "Shouldn't I know how I really feel?"

"Yes," I replied, "and I think you know how you really feel. You have mixed feelings. That is the feeling you have—*ambivalence*."

At this Brenda laughed. But she still felt that she should not have mixed feelings. She asked, "Shouldn't I know how I feel?" I countered that she does know her feelings—and they're mixed. We then talked about the fact that she has longtime friends about whom she has mixed feelings, which she accepts, and the possibility that the same thing is true with Mike.

"Maybe mixed feelings comes with knowing people," I offered.

"But if you love someone shouldn't you not have mixed feelings?"

"That sounds very idealistic. But unrealistic. *Maybe loving someone is accepting mixed feelings.* Maybe loving someone is seeing the bigger picture."

How do you think about your ambivalence? Do you have a set of rules about how you should feel? Check off any of the statements that apply to you:

- ☐ I should never have ambivalent feelings.

- ☐ If I am ambivalent, then I need to keep thinking about the issue to get rid of those mixed feelings.

- ☐ Other people can help me get rid of my ambivalence.

- ☐ I need to change anything that I feel ambivalent about.

- ☐ If I am ambivalent then I cannot make decisions.

- ☐ Only neurotic, anxious, and depressed people feel ambivalent.

- ☐ Almost everyone else is completely clear about the way they feel.

In which areas of your life do you have the most difficulty accepting ambivalence? In which areas is it easier to accept ambivalence?

_____

_____

_____

_____

_____

_____

_____

_____

When you feel ambivalent, do you think that you need to get rid of the ambivalence? Why?

_____

_____

_____

_____

_____

_____

_____

What would it mean to you if you could not get rid of mixed feelings? What if you had to live with these mixed feelings?

_____

_____

_____

_____

_____

_____

_____

If you think that you should not have mixed feelings, you will have difficulty tolerating them, living with, and accepting them. You will likely ruminate and worry about them, ask for reassurance, and have difficulty making decisions and living with the results of your decisions. You will be more prone to regret, looking back to the past and idealizing some alternative you did not choose. Your intolerance of mixed feelings may make you doubt the value of your daily life experiences and distract you from appreciating what you actually do have.

But what if you had a different view of ambivalence? What if you had more of the following thoughts and feelings about ambivalence?

Ambivalence is normal because all parts of life have ups and downs.

I can accept ambivalence rather than dwell on it.

Everything involves trade-offs.

Everyone has mixed feelings if they are honest with themselves.

I can make decisions with mixed feelings, because decisions always involve mixed feelings when you compare one alternative with another alternative.

Maximizers

A number of years ago I had lunch with a colleague in a diner. He studied the menu carefully. He turned to the waiter and began asking how the waiter would compare one entrée with another, going through about ten items. I found this irritating, and I am sure the waiter found it annoying as well. My colleague, who is a very intelligent person, was trying to make sure that he got the very best entrée, and he thought he needed to do all the comparisons.

Now this might seem like a rather trivial example (because it is), but imagine if you approach decisions in your life with the demand that you have to get the very best of everything. You won't settle for second place. It has to be the best. These folks are what psychologists refer to as *maximizers*. Maximizers are perfectionists when it comes to certain decisions. They won't settle for less. They keep searching and searching—for the perfect partner, the perfect job, the perfect friends. It's endless.

Well, that might sound like a good idea. But maximizing has its downside, which we touched on briefly in chapter 4. The research shows that maximizers take longer to make decisions, they require more information, they often search for irrelevant information, they find decision-making to be an unpleasant experience, and they are less satisfied with their choices. In fact, maximizers are more likely to experience regret after they have chosen something because they look back and wonder if there was something better at the time, or they think that there might be something better in the future (Schwartz et al. 2002; Parker, De Bruin, and Fischhoff 2007)

Mark's Story

Mark was a maximizer when it came to deciding to get married. He was in a long-term relationship with Deena, who he loved. He enjoyed her company and felt that their sex life was quite good. He told me that Deena was a kind, compassionate, forgiving person who was committed to him. He said he wanted to have children, and he thought that Deena would make a great mom.

But then there were the "buts." These included the fact that Deena was not as interested in business and politics as he was. He thought, "What if I get bored?" and then he worried, "What if someone else comes along who is better for me?" He acknowledged that Deena was by far the more desirable of all the women he ever dated. But he kept coming back to his complaints, his frustrations, his occasional boredom, and his fear that there was something better out there.

These were the assumptions that made Mark uncomfortable with his mixed feelings:

- I should never be bored in a relationship.

- I should keep focusing on the negative.

- I can't accept less than perfection in my partner.

- If I am ambivalent, it's a bad sign.

- I should keep searching until I am sure that there is no one better out there.

I pointed out to Mark that his maximizing, emotionally perfectionistic assumption that he should never be bored in a relationship was unrealistic. Boredom is just another transient emotion that we have about ourselves, our best friends, and the people we are intimate with. Why shouldn't we be occasionally bored in our interactions with people we love? Eventually Mark understood that boredom just comes with the territory.

Another assumption that Mark had, and which you may have as well, is that he had to continue to search for the best one out there. Let's think about this. There are about five and half billion people in the world. How likely is it that you will find the best one in the world? Not very likely. Does anyone have the best possible choice in the world? After all, you might think that your current partner is the best possible choice in the world, but have you "sampled" the other five and a half billion? No.

The Three Confusing C's: Clarity, Closure, and Certainty

Many of us have a mixed mind (no pun intended) when it comes to accepting ambivalence. That's because we're typically searching for clarity, closure, and certainty. We tend to believe that in finding these things we will have our answer. However, these elements are often elusive.

Clarity

You may think that accepting mixed feelings deprives you of the necessary clarity that you need about the way you "really feel" about what is important. You may equate clarity with the idea that there are no pros and cons. That isn't clarity—that's perfection. Maybe what is clear is that *there are pros and cons*. Maybe what is clear is that you have mixed feelings.

Let's take the metaphor of a rural area of New England where I have a house and where the weather is constantly changing. It could be sunny and 55 degrees one day, and it could be snowing and 20 degrees the next. The clouds come and go throughout the day. What is clear to me is that the weather changes, not that it is always sunny, always snowy, or always cloudy.

How can you have clarity if your experiences with your partner or your job or your friends are constantly changing? The idea of clarity is akin to thinking that you can take a snapshot of your life while your experiences and feelings change moment to moment each day. Clarity may be realizing that there is no clarity that is permanent or realistic.

Closure

You may think that by ruminating about your ambivalence—and constantly looking at the positives compared to the negatives—you will ultimately get closure. And in getting closure, you may believe it's the same as taking your feelings, perceptions, memories, and dreams and putting them in a box, closing it, and labeling it "done for." But our experiences are not like a box that you lock and store in an attic. You don't have an attic for memories.

Our experiences—all of them—are fluid, changing, unpredictable. Your life, memories, relationships, and past experiences of all kinds are part of an open book that you go back to, that can return to you at any time, that may be triggered by something you see or hear. There is no closure when life is an open book and all of what you experience is fluid, like the waves on a beach.

Sometimes those waves—your experiences—are mild, and sometimes they're strong. Watch the waves come and go. You don't have closure with an ocean that is constantly in motion.

Certainty

You may need or demand certainty because you equate uncertainty with a bad outcome. You may think that you have a responsibility to find certainty. But does uncertainty mean a bad outcome? I'm uncertain what the weather will be tomorrow but that doesn't mean that we will have a blizzard.

It may be difficult for you to tolerate doubts, especially when you think that you have to be able to predict the outcome with complete confidence. But there is no certainty in an uncertain world. The ocean keeps drifting, the waves crest and fall and rise again—unpredictability doesn't mean that you will drown if you ride the waves and accept the changing tides. After all, is there anything in your life that you have absolute certainty about? You don't know what the next person is going to say, how you will feel, whether your car will break down, or whether you will lose your job. In fact, if you had absolute certainty you would be bored with the complete predictability of everything. You might even begin to think that you have a need for uncertainty!

Choices

Even with your emotional perfectionism that leads you to seek clarity, closure, and certainty, you still can make a choice. You may think that you have no choice about ruminating about this ambivalence—no choice in whether you accept it or don't accept it. But this way of thinking is like equating ambivalence with the law of gravity on Earth: it's not a matter of how you look at it, it's *real* no matter what.

You may also believe that if you make a choice, you will likely regret it. You might think, "I will look back at my doubts and realize that I could have made another choice, and then I will really criticize myself." But keep in mind that maximizers who can't tolerate ambivalence are *more likely* to regret their decisions and the outcomes that they experience. So, if not tolerating uncertainty was the key issue, then maximizers would have less regret. But they don't. They have more regret.

What are the advantages of accepting ambivalence as a natural part of life—of relationships and of self-reflection?

_____

_____

_____

_____

_____

What if you thought of uncertainty as an inevitable part of lived experience? What if you accepted the idea that we can never know for sure what will happen?

_____

_____

_____

_____

In what areas of your life do you accept some uncertainty? Why?

_____

_____

_____

_____

What would be the advantage of giving up on clarity and embracing complexity and change instead?

_____

_____

_____

_____

_____

Problematic Strategies in Dealing with Ambivalence

Once you realize that you have mixed feelings, you might go off and running trying to cope with these feelings. When you are coping, you are likely trying to eliminate the mixed quality of your feelings to determine what you really feel—which, in your mind, should be only one way. In other words, you want your feelings to be either/or, black or white, in your mind.

There are a lot of ways that people cope with their feelings. Let's see how you handle your mixed feelings.

Which of the following do you do because you have difficulty accepting your mixed feelings? If the example does not apply to you, think of friends who have difficulty with their ambivalence and describe their experiences. Give examples.

Complaining: *You complain to other people or to the target of your mixed feelings about how you don't accept the downsides, the negatives, and the disappointments.*

_____

_____

_____

_____

_____

Collecting more and more information: *You think that you will be able to resolve your ambivalence by collecting more information, although your search for information often is biased toward the negative.*

_____

_____

_____

_____

_____

Always focusing on the negative and discounting the positive: *You tend to direct your attention toward the negatives to the exclusion of the positive, and filter things out that are positive. This makes you feel even more discouraged.*

_____

_____

_____

_____

_____

Seeking reassurance: *You seek reassurance that things will be okay—either from friends or the target of your ambivalence.*

_____

_____

_____

_____

_____

Ruminating: *You dwell on the fact that you have mixed feelings, turning things over and over in your mind so that you cannot simply live with ambivalence and enjoy the present moment.*

_____

_____

_____

_____

_____

Worrying that you will make the wrong decision: *You anticipate that you will make the wrong choice and later regret it.*

_____

_____

_____

_____

_____

Procrastinating: *You put off making decisions until you feel ready, passing up opportunities to either move forward or break off from something.*

_____

_____

_____

_____

_____

Hedging your bets: *You don't break off, because you have one foot in and one foot out.*

_____

_____

_____

_____

_____

Let's take a closer look at why some of these coping strategies are problematic:

☐ *Complaining* about your ambivalence will alienate people around you and keep you stuck in the negative. How can that help you?

☐ *Collecting more and more information* might make sense at first, but you might also be biased in the information that you collect—trying to prove your point or trying to eliminate your ambivalence. When do you know you have enough information?

☐ *Always focusing on the negative and discounting the positive* may lead you to overlook the good things that you already have.

☐ *Seeking reassurance* might work for a few minutes, but that won't eliminate mixed feelings since there may be good reasons to have mixed feelings. Reassurance doesn't change reality. Even if someone assures you of something positive, such as "You really love that person," it doesn't mean that your negative feelings won't return. Reassurance only feeds into your idea that you need to eliminate ambivalence—rather than own it, live with it, and normalize it.

☐ *Ruminating* about the future won't eliminate ambivalence, it will only make you depressed and anxious, which makes it harder to accept ambivalence.

☐ *Worrying* that you will make the wrong decision may be driven by your belief that worry will prepare you for the worst. But you end up living in a hypothetical world that may never actually exist—and it is always a negative world. In fact, chronic worry leads to depression.

☐ *Procrastinating* and putting off decisions keeps you frozen in your ambivalence and feeds into the perfectionistic idea that you cannot make decisions if you have mixed feelings. Indeed, decisions are about recognizing that you have mixed feelings but deciding to step forward anyway.

☐ *Hedging your bets* will only lead to minimizing your true capability and sabotaging your potential. If you have one foot in and one foot out, you will minimize your effectiveness.

To reiterate, the problem is that you don't accept that ambivalence is a legitimate emotional experience. You *can* have mixed feelings about someone or something, and those mixed feelings can be a completely realistic and honest way of experiencing things. It's not a problem. It's a realistic perception of what is going on.

So why not accept ambivalence?

The Myth of Pure Mind

People who believe in *pure mind* can't stand having mixed feelings, contradictory thoughts, unclarity, or unpleasant and unwanted emotions. It's like these experiences that we all have are a kind of stain on the purity of how things should be in your head. You think you have to be clear, consistent, and on top of things. You can't stand the noise, the fluidity of experience, the constantly changing information. You want everything in a little box, wrapped neatly, everything clear, concise, and coherent.

But that is not what reality is like. You are likely to notice mixed feelings at times about almost everything that is important to you: your partner, your best friend, your home, your job, where you live, your political and religious beliefs, and what you are watching on television. There is no pure mind, there is only a constantly changing set of experiences, perspectives, and feelings. It's like the music changes, but you still go on.

What if you abandoned the pure mind ideal? What if you accepted contradiction, confusion, and some illogical, unfair, unclear, and uncertain parts of existence? What is the payoff?

The payoff is that you don't have to be clear, you don't have to know for sure, you can accept incompleteness, and you can allow yourself the richness that comes from ambivalence. You can be more honest with yourself that you do, in fact, have mixed feelings at times. The payoff is that nothing needs to be perfect, there is no need for closure, you don't have to get to the bottom of things, and you don't need to find out how you really feel.

You can simply acknowledge honestly, confidently: *I guess I have mixed feelings about that.* And that is an honest answer. That is *the* answer. You have mixed feelings. Case closed.

Tradeoffs Come with the Territory

One of the difficulties that many people have is what I call "existential perfectionism"—that is, the belief that important things in their lives should be free from any downside. The existential perfectionist wants that perfect relationship, dream job, and place to live. This is the Utopian view—the view that there is a nirvana just around the corner. (By the way, the word "utopia" is Latin for "no place." As someone joked years ago, "Utopia is a small town in upstate New York, but no one lives there anymore.")

When it comes to the real world of relationships, jobs, and places to live, there is no Utopia, there is no dream that lasts as an ideal, there is no place or person without some downside. Everything has a cost. Let's take marriage. Marriage has its benefits, but it has its downsides at times. You and your partner will have disagreements, you will realize that you don't have complete freedom anymore, you have to accommodate someone else, and you may incur financial costs that you didn't expect. But maybe it's worth the cost. The positives may include stability, having someone to share things with, and building a life together.

Everything eventually involves upsides and downsides. There is no free lunch. Certain things come with the territory. For instance, your job may occasionally involve boring, unpleasant work with long hours. But it may also be a means of support, personal and professional growth, and eventual advancement.

I live in New York City, which is expensive, noisy, and crowded. But it is also one of the greatest cities to live in, with museums, interesting people, a wide range of ethnic restaurants, and so on. Tradeoffs involve positives and negatives.

Everything has tradeoffs. If you want to be married, you have to accept certain tradeoffs. If you want to work, there will be things you won't like. And wherever you live, there will be pros and cons. The issue is not only "What is the dream?" but "What tradeoffs are you willing to accept?"

Let's examine the tradeoffs you have in various aspects of your life. On the worksheet that follows, list positive and negative examples for each life domain. Then quantify the pros and cons using a percentage scale that adds up to 100 percent. For example, you might rate the pros and cons of work as evenly split, 50-50. But you might rate friendships as 70-30. In the far-right column, subtract the negative from the positive. For example, if the positives of your current relationship are 60 and the negatives are 40, then the resulting positive-negative is +20.

Examining Tradeoffs

Life Domain	Positives	%	Negatives	%	Positive-Negative
Committed Relationship					
Being on My Own					
Friendships					
Work					
Where I Live					
Health and Fitness					
Other:					

Do most areas of your life have both positives and negatives? What does that tell you?

_____

_____

_____

_____

What do you make of the fact that nothing is completely positive and nothing is completely negative?

_____

_____

_____

_____

Which positives and which negatives are most important to you?

_____

_____

_____

_____

Which negatives do you think can improve? How can they improve?

_____

_____

_____

_____

_____

Do other people also have these positives and negatives? What do you make of that? How do they deal with that?

_____

_____

_____

_____

What if we thought of tradeoffs as part of the richness and complexity of real life? What if we thought of them as things that simply come with the territory?

_____

_____

_____

_____

Keep in mind that while there may be certain qualities in every life domain that are really appealing to you, they may come with characteristics that you may find challenging at times. For example, Laura complained that her partner, Jeff, was not emotionally tuned in to her and that he seemed to focus too much on being practical. When I asked her what she liked about him when they were first getting involved, she said that he was reliable, hardworking, and level-headed. So, certain things come with the territory, and what you don't like now may be the flip side of what you liked (or will like) in a different context or time.

The Symphony

What if we think of our emotions as notes in a musical score? If we can't tolerate ambivalence then we would want everything to be simple and clear—and the musical score would consist of one note repeated over and over. Sounds monotonous to me. But what if we think of our feelings as a symphony with different movements, notes contrasting with one another, sounds supplementing each other, notes going up and down, fast and slow? Now, that is music.

Let's take your mixed feelings about your friends. If you are honest with yourself, you know that there are things about them that you don't like, things that you find especially annoying. Yet there are many things that you do like. So now you are aware of a wide range of honest feelings you have about your friendships. Imagine that each of these feelings—positive, negative, and neutral—is a different note, a different part of this symphony. The music is sometimes soft, sometimes loud, sometimes fast, sometimes slow. It's all part of the bigger experience. All of it is part of friendship: the good and the bad and the neutral. Just listen to the symphony—all the notes, all the movements.

How would it help you if you thought of your experiences as symphonies with many notes, contrasting sounds, and different movements?

Take-Home Points

♦ Notice whether you are having difficulty accepting ambivalence.

♦ Notice whether you accept mixed feelings in certain areas of your life.

♦ Open to the idea that mixed feelings come from the complexity of life rather than a signal that there is something wrong that needs to be fixed.

♦ Notice whether ambivalence makes it difficult for you to tolerate any negatives, adds to your general dissatisfaction, makes you more indecisive, or makes you more regretful.

♦ Consider that searching for clarity, closure, and certainty are impossible tasks.

♦ Maybe ambivalence is not the problem. Maybe the problem is that you think ambivalence is the problem.

♦ There is no pure mind. Our minds are more like a kaleidoscope. Often we have conflicting feelings about the same thing.

♦ Look for a relative balance rather than an experience with no tradeoffs.

♦ Think of experiences like you would a symphony: many notes, many movements, many changes.

CHAPTER 9

What Do I Care About?

If you are like a lot of people, you may realize that what upset you in the past doesn't seem so important today. Your feelings might change within an hour, a week, or a year. For example, you might get extremely angry in traffic, start driving aggressively, and scare your passengers. But an hour later you might realize that it wasn't worth it to get so angry, that it didn't really matter that you were delayed five minutes. You might even wonder why you cared what someone in another car thought about you.

As we learned in chapters 1 and 2, our emotions often tell us that something is very important, essential, or true. For example, loneliness tells us that being connected is important. Yet, we have also learned that at other times our emotions may mislead us—may make something seem important that, in the long journey of our lives, is not really that important. *What seems important now may not be important later.*

In this chapter, you will clarify what is truly of value—what is important—to you. You'll also learn how to direct yourself toward a life that you will feel is worth the struggle. The exercises in this chapter will give you insights and direction, especially in determining when your emotions are misleading you to think that something is important when really it's only of passing concern. Keeping the bigger picture in mind can help you cope with your emotions—and, in some cases, reveal what your larger goals truly are.

So, what is important?

Looking Back from the End

You may be familiar with Tolstoy's story, *The Death of Ivan Ilyich*. Ivan was a careful, obedient government worker who always tried to be dutiful. But then he learns that he has a terminal illness. As Ivan is lying in his bed, he hears family members and friends in another room going about their daily business. It's as if his death will be a momentary inconvenience and everything else will go on. He wonders what his life was really about. Did he really love the people he loved, did he grow in any meaningful way, did he make his life and those of others an important priority?

A number of years ago, I was talking with a man who told me that his father had died five years earlier after an illness. I commented, "Was that a hard time for you?" He said, "Yes, it was the hardest time during that year when I took care of him. But, you know, it was the best year of my life. We got to talk, I told him how much I loved him, and he told me how much I mattered to him. We grew closer than we ever had. It was a sad time, but it was also an important time for me."

When people are approaching the end of their lives they may fear death, fear leaving people behind, and fear the sorrow that others will experience. But their regrets often include not telling people they loved them, realizing when it is too late what was really important. They may often regret harsh words said or not being there for their kids. They regret not forgiving people.

One man told me that people should go to more funerals. I asked him why and he said, "I went to a funeral last week. It seems that at my age there are more of those, but it made me think. People got up and spoke about what they remembered about this man who died. His kids spoke, his wife spoke, I spoke. And what I realized is that we remember the personal touch, the fun things that we shared, his acts of kindness, his humor."

So, I want you to think about what you would want people to say about you at your funeral. How do you want to be remembered? What will people think was important about knowing you, about having you in their lives? Do you want people to remember you for your success, your accomplishments, your appearance? For the things that you own or the things that you were always right about? Do you want them to remember you for your kindness, your laughter, your ability to make others laugh? Do you want them to remember the times they shared with you, how you lifted them up, how you forgave them when they fell down, how you were the one they could count on?

I know it's sad to think about the end, but we will all face it. The good news is that you can start building your values, personal qualities, and connections with the people you care about so that, from now until that time in the distant future, you will live according to the values that will make your life a life worth living, a life worth sharing.

Imagine you are observing your own funeral. What do you want people to say about you? Why is that important?

_____

_____

_____

_____

_____

Now that you have thought about what you want people to remember you for, what can you do this week that is aligned with those values?

_____

_____

_____

_____

The Power of Negation

Most of us realize at times that we take a lot for granted. But sometimes this realization comes too late. This exercise is one that can help clarify what is important to you and why it is important to you. It's based on the power of *negation* to affirm what matters. If we take it away, what would you miss?

Take It All Away

Close your eyes and imagine that you have disappeared. You have no body, no senses, no memory, no possessions, no relationships. You have been reduced to nothing. You have disappeared.

Now, imagine that you can get one thing back at a time. You don't know how many things you will get back, but in order to get anything back you have to convince a supreme power (whatever that might be to you) that this one thing is important to you. You have to make a case for why you are grateful, why you want it back, why you need it.

For now, just think about what you would want back first. Why?

Beth's Story

I shared the idea of negation with Beth, who was feeling down because her boss was making another unreasonable demand of her. Beth was angry and wanted to tell him off. It made sense that she felt this way, but getting into a power struggle would only make matters worse. Because of her anger, it seemed that the rest of her life had lost its importance, its texture, its meaning for her.

So we tried the negation exercise, and I asked her what she wanted back. "I guess the first thing I want back is my daughter, Donna." Why? "Because I love her. She means everything to me. I know that we have had some difficult times, but she is really the center of my life. We have been through so much together."

I replied, "Okay, you have made a case, you can have Donna. What else would you want back?"

Beth said, "I want my eyesight. I want to see. Seeing Donna is at the top of my list. But I also want to see the sky, the trees, I want to see my friends, I want to see the ocean, the beach."

I said, "So, there is a lot to see. What else would you want back?"

"I want my hearing. I want to hear my daughter, I want to hear her voice. I want to hear music." As Beth went through each thing that she wanted back, her mood improved.

I said, "You know, you didn't ask for anything related to work, nothing about money, nothing about possessions. What do you make of this?"

Donna then realized that those things—work, money, possessions—were not the most important things in her life.

When we are upset about something, when we are angry, we don't notice the things that truly matter to us. In fact, the things most important to most of us are typically right in front of us almost every day. We just need to notice them.

Imagine everything has been taken away and you are nothing. You no longer exist. But you can get one thing back at a time. You don't know how many things you will be allowed to get back, but in order to get something back you need to make a convincing case that it matters to you, that you appreciate it. What do you want back and why is it important to you? Name five things and write down why each is important to you.

_____

_____

_____

_____

_____

_____

_____

In the past, you have gotten upset about things that happened or that you worried about. Were any of these things on your list of what you wanted back? Why or why not?

_____

_____

_____

_____

_____

Become the Person You Admire

The ancient Greeks described "flourishing" as the key to a fulfilling life. Flourishing meant a sense of happiness and meaningfulness in living according to your values. Aristotle described certain qualities of character as the source of happiness and flourishing, and suggested that we will feel more connected with wisdom if we find the balance of these values (he called them *virtues)*. These included courage, truthfulness, patience, modesty, friendliness, and other qualities. Aristotle proposed that it was the proper *balance* of each quality that constituted the right level. For example, too much courage constituted rashness, while too little was cowardice. Too much patience meant a lack of spirit or energy, while too little led to being easily upset. Too much modesty meant shyness, while too little modesty equated shamelessness.

Christianity's virtues include charity, diligence, patience, kindness, and humility, and in Hinduism we find freedom from anger, control over your senses, non-stealing, and truthfulness. Buddhism recognizes loving-kindness, compassion, joy for others and for the self, and treating all beings equally. You may have your own preferences of values and virtues.

One way to identify values and virtues is to imagine the kind of person you admire. Do you admire someone who is hostile, angry, vindictive, or deceptive? Or do you admire someone who is flexible, agreeable, forgiving, or honest? Do you admire kindness and consideration? We can think about our values for ourselves as those qualities that we admire in someone else. And we can direct our behavior—as much as possible—to become the person that we admire.

Choosing behaviors that are guided by your values might mean that you don't always go along with what other people are doing; for example, if you value fairness toward people who are less fortunate, then you might not tolerate listening to someone tell a racist joke. It might mean that you don't always act on your immediate and powerful emotions; for instance, if you value your commitment to your partner, then you might not pursue a one-night stand with someone else. It might mean that you think about practicing self-control (temperance), kindness, forgiveness, and compassion toward other people and toward yourself—if those are your values.

Think of some of the qualities that you admire in other people. Check to see that those characteristics are listed in the left column; if not, feel free to add them. In the second column, use a 0 to 6 scale to indicate how important that value is to you. In the far-right column, indicate how well you think you are achieving that value in your life using the academic scale from A to F, whereby A corresponds to excellent and F corresponds to failing. We are interested in what is important to you and how you are living according to your goals and values. There are no scores or cutoff points. This is about setting goals and reaching them. Are you leading a life consistent with your values and reaching your goals?

Which Values Are Important to Me?

Scale:

1 = not at all important to me

2 = somewhat unimportant to me

3 = slightly unimportant of me

4 = slightly important to me

5 = somewhat important to me

6 = very important to me

Value	How Important Is This to Me? (scale of 0–6)	How Am I Doing? (scale of A–F)
Courage		
Truthfulness		
Patience		
Modesty		
Charity		
Diligence		

Kindness		
Humility		
Freedom from anger		
Control over my senses		
Respect for others' property and rights		
Joy for others		
Compassion		
Treating others equally		
Other:		
Other:		
Other:		

How are you doing living according to your most important values? How would your life be different if you made those a real priority on a daily basis? If something is important to you—for example, being a good friend—but you score low (for example, you give yourself a D), think about what you can do to improve to live according to this value. For example, how could you be a better friend?

_____

_____

_____

_____

_____

_____

Let's look at Ron, who has often been irritable with his wife, Beverly. Ron has been hijacked by his anger, leading to significant conflicts with Beverly. Ron sinks into guilty sadness feeling that he is ruining his relationship. After Ron completed the worksheet "Which Values Are Important to Me?" he realized that he wanted to develop more patience, kindness, freedom from anger, and compassion. He wanted to be more aligned with these values when dealing with not only Beverly but his two children, his brother, and the people he works with.

Using the next worksheet, "Actions Consistent with My Values," Ron kept track of positive actions for a week. For example, he waited patiently while Beverly talked about her day, he showed kindness and compassion when she told him about her disagreements with her mother, and he refrained from criticizing her. He also showed patience with one of his colleagues, showing kindness in telling her that he knew that she was trying and that sometimes things took a while. He helped an elderly woman cross the street and wished her a good day. As Ron focused more on the virtues, values, and strengths that were important to him, he began feeling less irritable. He realized that he was on his way to becoming the person he admires.

Every day is an opportunity to move in the right direction. So let's practice right now and for the next few days! Use the following worksheet to note the specific actions you took each day to live in accordance with your values. In the first column, list all the values, virtues, or strengths that are important to you; if you need help, you can refer to those you rated a 5 or 6 on the worksheet "Which Values Are Important to Me." In the other columns, write down any actions you took on two separate days. Make a copy of this worksheet, or download it from http://www.newharbinger.com/44802, to extend this exercise over several more days.

Actions Consistent with My Values

Important Values	Date: _____ **Actions I Took Today**	Date: _____ **Actions I Took Today**

How would you feel if you did more things more often that are consistent with the values that are important to you? How would your life be better?

_____

_____

_____

_____

_____

What gets in the way of acting in accordance with your values?

_____

_____

_____

_____

What can you do differently this week to expand your behavior that would be consistent with your values?

_____

_____

_____

_____

_____

Values and the Roles We Play

All of us have different roles we play in our lives. You may be a mother, sister, brother, father, husband, wife, partner, son, daughter, friend, caretaker, worker, boss, neighbor, member of a religious community, pet owner, volunteer, or some other role. Some of these roles are more important to us than others. Many roles involve other people, which is why we sometimes have difficulty in our relationships with certain individuals.

So, how would this work if your goal, based on your values, was to be a better partner? Let's look at Ron's list of targets to be a better husband:

- Don't criticize.

- Don't label.

- Try to see her point of view.

- Be more patient.

- Compliment her more.

- Be forgiving.

- Let go of past resentments.

- Plan some fun things.

- Show affection.

- Be appreciative.

We can come up with a list of actions to be better in our roles in other life domains just as well. The goal is to target behaviors that are consistent with our values, to become the person we admire. Now it's your turn to see how you can commit to valued action.

Think of the different roles that you play in your life. On the worksheet that follows, review the various common roles; if you do not see a role listed, add it. Next, list whatever valued actions you can take this week to be better in that role. For example, next to the role of friend, you might write down that you will contact a friend, ask how they are doing, compliment them, and then schedule something fun to do together. Then, after a week, return to this worksheet and, in the third column, record whether you were able to follow through on your valued action. Either way, keep focusing on acting toward your valued goals on a daily basis.

Valued Actions for Important Roles

Important Roles for Me	Valued Actions Toward Goals	How Did I Do?
Romantic partner		
Parent		
Sibling		
Son or daughter		
Worker		
Colleague		
Neighbor		
Volunteer		
Other:		
Other:		

Take-Home Points

♦ Your values are important to you and they determine your emotions.

♦ Think about what you would like people to say about you at your funeral. Then try to become the person that they describe.

♦ Imagine that everything has been taken away from you, but you can get one thing back at a time if you make a strong case for it. Think about would you want back and how you appreciate it.

♦ Focus on becoming the person you admire.

♦ Consider the different roles that you play and how you can include valued action in each one.

♦ Practice valued action each day.

CHAPTER 10

The Worst Ways to Cope

When we feel overwhelmed by intense feelings, we often act or think impulsively and jump to old habits, problematic behaviors, and self-destructive strategies. In this chapter we will review some of the most common problematic strategies for coping and look at the advantages and disadvantages of each one. You will learn to choose what you think is in your long-term best interests.

Problematic Coping Strategies

Your goal is to build a life worth living. A long life, a full life, a life that goes beyond the present moment. The goal is not to feel better for the next five minutes. The goal is to feel better for the next five years. The long term is more important than the short term. Building this life will mean identifying and changing your unhelpful ways of coping. It won't be easy at times, but the objective is to do the hard things now, so life is easier in the future.

So, let's get started.

Alcohol and Drugs

There's an old saying that "There is no problem that drinking won't make worse." The same with drugs. I've never known anyone whose goal was to have an alcohol or drug problem. Have you? We tend to have great confidence that we can handle things—especially if they make us feel better over the next five minutes. But certain things can spiral out of control and rob us of living a valued life.

What are the signs of a drinking or drug problem? The National Institute of Alcoholism and Alcohol Abuse recommends asking the following questions to assess whether you (or a loved) one may have Alcohol Use Disorder. The same questions can be modified for drug abuse.

In the past year, have you:

☐ Had times when you ended up drinking more or longer than you intended?

☐ More than once wanted to cut down or stop drinking, or tried to, but couldn't?

☐ Spent a lot of time drinking? Or being sick or getting over the aftereffects?

☐ Experienced craving—a strong need or urge to drink?

☐ Found that drinking—or being sick from drinking—often interfered with taking care of your home or family? Or caused job troubles? Or school problems?

☐ Continued to drink even though it was causing trouble with your family or friends?

☐ Given up or cut back on activities that were important or interesting to you, or gave you pleasure, in order to drink?

☐ More than once gotten into situations while or after drinking that increased your chances of getting hurt (such as driving, swimming, using machinery, walking in a dangerous area, or having unsafe sex)?

☐ Continued to drink even though it was making you feel depressed or anxious or adding to another health problem? Or after having had a memory blackout?

☐ Had to drink much more than you once did to get the effect you wanted? Or found that your usual number of drinks had much less effect than before?

☐ Found that when the effects of alcohol were wearing off, you had withdrawal symptoms, such as trouble sleeping, shakiness, irritability, anxiety, depression, restlessness, nausea, or sweating? Or sensed things that were not there?

Alcohol and drug abuse and dependence are significant problems for many people with emotional difficulties. It is easy to minimize your problem and convince yourself that you have everything under control. I am not saying that people need to abstain—although some people do need to abstain. But it is essential to look at how you use alcohol and other drugs to manage your moods. Keep in mind that alcohol is a central nervous system depressant, which means that, over the long term, you will likely become depressed and even more anxious.

Many people feel controlled by the addicted part of their brain that sends out messages about craving, needing a drink or a fix, and minimizing the problem. Think about the *permission-giving thoughts* that you have about alcohol and drugs. You might say to yourself, "I can handle another drink," "There are people worse off than I am," "I deserve it since I had a bad day," or "I just want to celebrate having a good day." But if you have a drinking problem and you are listening to your permission-giving thoughts, then you will end up reinforcing your problem. Your "solution" is now the problem.

It's beyond the scope of this book to help treat your alcohol or drug abuse problem. If you believe you may have a problem with addiction, seek help from a qualified counselor. Millions of people give up drinking and drugs to get a better handle on their emotions. And they are taking back their lives—one day at a time.

Binge Eating

Eating disorders should be called "emotional-eating disorders," since they often involve problematic behaviors to cope with emotions. If you are feeling anxious and lonely, you may find yourself bingeing on sweets, carbohydrates, or anything that is available that fills you up. You are stuffing down those feelings, distracting yourself from your emotions, and adding another problem. You might follow your bingeing with purging—vomiting, using laxatives, or even excessive exercise.

You can learn more about coping with binge eating and purging by reading the excellent guide by Christopher Fairburn (2013), *Overcoming Binge Eating: The Proven Program to Learn Why You Binge and How You Can Stop*. You can also seek professional counseling from a therapist who specializes in cognitive behavioral therapy for eating disorders.

Complaining

One of the key elements of being a human being is complaining about things. We complain about the weather, our boss, our friends, and anything bad that happens to us. And we also complain about things that are not happening to us, for example, we complain about what we watch on television, read online, or hear that people have done.

Complaining may help us find that others agree with us, that our perceptions and feelings are validated, and that our feelings make sense. And complaining may even help us feel that we are bonding with others as we take turns listening to each other's complaints.

But our complaining can also turn into rumination that we may inadvertently dump on friends and family. This kind of persistent, negative focus can initially lead to supportive comments like, "It will get better" or "I know how you feel" or "Maybe you can try this or that." However, chronic complaining can involve our rejection of any supportive comments. For example, Rachel complained about her brother, who complained to her about his relationship with his wife. When I suggested that maybe his marriage was hard for him and that he might be depressed, Rachel got angry with me, saying, "You don't understand what it is like to have to listen to him!" Sometimes our complaining leads to *help rejection*, whereby we may point out things that are negative and then get angry when the listener tries to be helpful.

We get so focused on the negative things that are happening to us—or what we are thinking about—that we just go on and on. The other person tries to be supportive, but then we reject their advice or help. They then feel that we don't want to hear their point of view, and so they begin to withdraw. Then we get depressed because our support network is falling apart. This pattern of complaining, help rejection, and withdrawal of social support is a major predictor of depression (Joiner, Brown, and Kistner 2006).

Getting support and having people hear what you say can be a difficult balance, since you don't want to get hijacked by your negativity with your friends. But it is important to be able to share your feelings—even your complaints. Here are some guidelines for how to share your feelings without driving people away:

- **Edit down what you say.** Don't go on and on. Otherwise, the other person might feel overwhelmed and begin to tune out. Limit what you say to short bites—two minutes at a time at most. This gives the other person a chance to take part in the conversation.

- **Give the other person a chance to talk.** Don't interrupt them, don't talk over them.

- **Don't attack the listener.** If you want to share your feelings, then you have to allow them to agree or disagree. If you attack people who support you, then you jeopardize your support.

- **Validate the validator.** Let them know that you appreciate their support. You can say, "I know I am complaining" or "I know this may sound negative at times," and add, "But I want you to know that I appreciate your support and I know it's not always easy to give the support."

- **Share positives as well as negatives.** Don't just focus on the negatives. This accomplishes two things: it breaks up the stream of negativity so that you don't sound consistently negative, and it also gets you to think about positives to put things in perspective.

- **Describe a solution when you describe a problem.** For example, if you complain about being lonely, you can also interject that you are signing up for some activities with other people. This shifts you into problem-solving mode, not just complaining mode.

- **Don't sound like your own worst enemy.** Avoid continual self-criticism, since this will only add to your low self-esteem. Rather than making global statements about yourself that are negative ("I am such a loser") you can make specific statements about a mistake and then what you learned from it ("I made a bad choice to spend time with him, but I think I have learned something from it about what is good for me and what isn't").

- **Respect advice.** Respect what people say, even when you don't like it. You can say, "I will have to think about what you said, because right now I am not sure if that would work for me, so I need to stand back and give it time. But I do appreciate your support because I know you are trying to be helpful."

Seeking Reassurance

Social support can often be a great way for us to reduce stress. Consider yourself fortunate if you have someone who can validate you, listen to your thoughts and feelings, and help you put things in perspective. But sometimes social support can lead to excessive complaining, such as when you start talking about something that might happen or has happened, and then you go on and on.

Another way that seeking reassurance can be problematic is if you continually turn to others to ask, "Am I going to be okay?" or "Should I do this or that?" Doing so too often may undermine your own ability to make decisions. For example, Carlos, who was suffering from fears of contamination (he had obsessive-compulsive disorder), would ask me if he was going to be okay if he touched various objects. This reassurance seeking became another compulsion for him. Carlos didn't think he could do these things without my telling him he was going to be okay. I told him that getting over his fear of contamination involved not getting continual reassurance. He had to make his own decision, face his fears, and accept the uncertainty about contamination.

You probably realize that reassurance from someone else is not really going to solve your problem. And you likely know that you can always discount their reassurance based on the fact that they don't know any better than you do what is going to work or what will happen. It's not reassurance you need, it's the willingness to do things that are uncomfortable and make the decisions that are hard to make. It's facing the uncertainty that is needed.

Be honest with yourself and ask whether you might be better off if you reduced the degree to which you seek reassurance. You simply need to find the right balance.

Avoiding Uncomfortable Situations

One of the hallmarks of anxiety and depression is that we often avoid people, places, and things that make us uncomfortable. Sometimes this makes sense—for example, if you don't need to interact with someone who is hostile or abusive, it is better to avoid them. Or if you are trying to cut back on drinking, and your friends want to take you to a bar where they will get blasted, it might be better to decline the invitation. Avoidance can be selective and adaptive, so you need to think about making choices that are in your best interest.

However, we can't always avoid situations that make us uncomfortable. For example, if you are at school or at work, you cannot easily avoid running into people that push your buttons. You cannot easily avoid news in the media that might be upsetting. And you cannot always avoid unpredictable situations or stimuli that elicit strong feelings, such as hearing a song at a restaurant that might remind you of a traumatic experience from the past.

The problem with avoidance is that we maintain our fear of what originally upset us. We don't learn when it is safe or that we can do difficult things and survive. Because we use avoidance to gain "safety," we never feel really safe in certain situations. We never learn that we can tolerate difficult emotions and difficult situations, and that we *can* survive. As we avoid and pull the wagons around us, our world becomes smaller and smaller.

Think of avoidance like riding a bicycle with training wheels for your entire life. You never learn that you don't need the extra wheels.

You *will* need to face difficult memories, unpleasant feelings, and difficult people. you can't live in a cocoon. Life keeps coming at you, and you can't always duck out of the way.

So, what is the answer? *You have to go through it to get past it.*

Eloise's Story

Eloise told me that she was in the building that got hit by one of the planes on 9/11. She ran from the building, thinking that she was going to die any second. Her trauma was real and her feelings made sense. Soon after, she became afraid of any plane in the sky, and she feared going into the subways because she worried about another attack. Eloise would wake in terror from disaster nightmares that seemed real. She began arranging her life around avoidance, drinking to calm her pain, and avoiding going out. As she became more depressed, her anxiety seemed to be more easily triggered by images, sounds, people, and ordinary events.

We worked for several months on expanding her ability to confront the experiences and memories that she avoided. First, we started with Eloise forming an image of the plane in the sky. Her anxiety rose and she felt more afraid, but as we stayed with the image for a while her anxiety began to subside. Eloise felt safe in my office. Then I asked her to form an image of the plane flying slowly sideways and to imagine that she controlled the movement of the plane. She imagined it flying backward, slowly, and then going up and down. This gave her a sense of control, and her anxiety began to decrease.

We listed a number of situations that made her anxious—the subway, walking outside when there was a plane overhead—and over a few weeks she began to take more chances. Each challenge made Eloise anxious, but as she confronted her fears her anxiety would decrease. Even when it didn't decrease as quickly as she would wish, she at least felt some sense of empowerment that she had faced her fears. Her sleep improved and she decreased her drinking. She began seeing friends more often. Eventually, Eloise went downtown to where the buildings had been bombed and walked around the area for thirty minutes. It was hard. She initially didn't think she could do it, but she did.

Eloise felt her fear, faced it, and went through it. She got past it.

WHAT ARE YOU AVOIDING?

Think about the situations, people, and places that you currently avoid. Yes, it's hard, because you can't stand thinking about them. They make you feel so bad. Maybe it's the memory of a past relationship, or a recollection of someone criticizing you, or the loss of someone you loved. You say, "I can't think about it, it's too upsetting." So, you cut that out of your life.

Kevin avoided going to the part of the university campus where he and Linda had spent a lot of time before their breakup. As a result of his avoidance, he had cut himself off from his friends and the memory of their relationship. I asked him what thoughts he had when he thought about going back into that place. Kevin sadly said, "I remember we seemed so happy, and then it ended, and then I felt so depressed."

And what did the breakup mean to him? Kevin paused and reflected: "I could never be happy again without Linda." We explored this belief that Linda could be the only source of his happiness, and he began to realize that he had been quite happy before Linda and that he and Linda had a lot of difficulties. In fact, there were times that he had thought of breaking up with Linda.

Using the worksheet that follows, list some of the people, places, memories, and situations that you currently avoid. In the second column, describe what actually happened that makes it hard to face. In the third column, list the thoughts you have that make these experiences so difficult.

Coping with Avoidance

What Do You Avoid?	Why? What Happened?	What Upsetting Thoughts Do You Have?
People		
Places		
Memories		
Situations		
Other:		

Develop a plan to gradually confront situations and people that you have been avoiding. Begin by imagining being in the presence of the people or places that you avoid. Imagine tolerating them. Then, if possible, you can engage in exposure to the situations—gradually, slowly, maybe not completely. You can get close, step away, try again several times. You can see if you can tolerate what seems difficult and unpleasant.

I tried exposure exercises with Kevin, who had been avoiding places that reminded him of Linda. He started with imagery—tolerating the picture in his mind of being in the building where Linda had been with him. This brought back sad and anxious feelings. But as we repeated this exercise, and as he eventually physically went to the area where they had spent time, he realized that the wave of uncomfortable feelings would pass, that he could get through it and past it—even though it was hard to do. He discovered that exposure was worth doing.

It was like taking back part of his life.

Ruminating and Worrying

A common response to difficult emotions is to dwell on the negative. Rumination is the continual focus on negative thoughts to the extent that they never seem to leave. It's not simply the occurrence of a negative thought, since that can be a momentary event for you that you can let go of. No, rumination is the persistence of the negative thought—like an unpleasant visitor who shows up and stays well past their welcome. People who are prone to rumination are more likely to get depressed and stay depressed and, unfortunately, women are much more likely to ruminate than men (Nolen-Hoeksema, Parker, and Larson 1994; Papageorgiou and Wells 2001a; Papageorgiou and Wells 2001b; Well and Papageorgiou 2004).

So, why do we ruminate and worry? What do we hope to gain from dwelling on something?

There are a number of "very good reasons" that you might have to ruminate and worry:

- You may think you have no choice—it's simply that the thought pops into your head and you are off and running. You are hijacked. You experience the rumination as a mental wave that crashes over you and takes you away.

- You may think that you will get the answer to your question ("Why is this happening to me?" or "Why did she say that?"), and this will reduce the uncertainty that you can't stand.

- You may think that the rumination will help you solve a problem—so that these bad things won't happen to you and you will be rid of this rumination forever—or, at least, for a while.

- You may think that the rumination will motivate you, keep you on your toes, and get you inspired to make things better.

- You may think that you need to be responsible all the time. You may believe that if something bad occurs in your imagination then you have a responsibility to deal with it. For example, if you have a thought that something bad can happen to your child, you may think that you have a responsibility to worry about it in order to make sure it doesn't happen.

- You may think that by worrying about something you can avoid being surprised—you will be prepared for the worst, because you have rehearsed it and it won't be that surprising to you.

Let's look at these "very good reasons" for dwelling on the negative and see if there is an alternative. Let's take the "mental hijack"—the belief that an intrusive thought necessarily has to carry you away. Imagine that you are at work and you are dwelling on a negative thought that has popped into your head. Your boss interrupts you and says, "I need to talk to you about this project we are working on." Do you ever say, "I'm sorry, I can't talk to you right now because I am currently busy worrying about something in the future"? Of course you don't. You allow yourself to get interrupted. And interruptions often pull you away from your worry, and you don't bother going back to it.

So, what if you intentionally interrupted your worry and set aside an appointment with your worry? Let's call this "worry time." This is a specific time when you will address whatever worries and ruminations you have had at other points in the day or night. Try it for fifteen minutes during the day at whatever time will work best for you.

Worry time will allow you to break away from the hijack of your intrusive thoughts, get on with your life in some positive ways, and get around to your worries at a time when you will really focus on them. Now, many of my clients say, "That's impossible—I have no control!" But I have found that almost everyone is able to set aside some worries until later—much to their surprise—which frees up a lot of time for living their lives.

So, what time of the day during the next week can you set aside fifteen minutes to focus on your worry? Commit to a time: _____. Then make a copy of the following worksheet (or download and print copies from http://www.newharbinger.com/44802) and fill it out every day for the next week.

Worry Time

Each day when you have a worry, jot it down here and set it aside for worry time. You can say, "Okay, that's a worry and I will get around to it later."

Worry 1: _____

_____

Worry 2: _____

_____

Worry 3: _____

_____

Worry 4: _____

_____

Worry 5: _____

_____

During worry time, set a timer for fifteen minutes. Then go through your list of worries from earlier in the day, starting with the first one.

How do you feel about the worry right now? Does it bother you as much now? Why or why not?

_____

_____

_____

_____

Will it be productive for you to worry about this right now? Will worrying lead to something you can do today to make progress on the thing you're worrying about? Specifically, what is it you can do?

_____

_____

_____

_____

Or will it be unproductive to worry about this right now? That is, is there anything you can do today to make progress on solving this problem? Yes or no?

_____

_____

If dwelling on this matter is unproductive, what would be the advantages of accepting uncertainty right now? What would be the disadvantages? Specify.

Advantages: _____

_____

_____

Disadvantages: _____

_____

_____

What limitations could you accept right now?

_____

_____

_____

Blaming Other People

We often find ourselves dwelling on our anger and resentment in blaming other people for our feelings. Do any of these statements sound familiar? "The reason I am angry is that my partner doesn't listen to me," "The reason I drink so much is that my partner is so critical," or "The reason that I am depressed is that my parents didn't love me."

Certainly, it is true that other people are often part of our problem. How our parents treated us—especially how they responded to our feelings when we were kids—is an important part of what we are like today. And if your partner or close friends treat you poorly, you have a legitimate point that conflict, misunderstanding, and criticism can be part of your difficulty. But how far and for how long do you go with your blaming? Are you getting hijacked by your belief that your emotional difficulties are entirely caused by someone else?

I often will see a husband come into therapy because his wife has told him he has to get help for his anger. Seldom does this kind of client say, "I have an anger problem." What he is really saying is, "My wife makes me angry." And what he would really like to say is, "She is the one with the problem, why isn't she here? I don't want to be here and I don't need to be here." This is a version of "the problem is my partner," which is a good predictor of continued conflict.

The problem with blaming other people for our feelings is that it leads us to believe that we can do nothing to change the way we feel. We think that it's up to the other person to change, and, of course, they are completely out of our control. We usually can't change other people, we can't change the past, and we can't get our parents to undo what they said or did years ago. So, while blaming others can give us a sense of being right—of being morally self-righteous—it only makes us feel as if there is nothing we can do.

Sharon's Story

Sharon had spent four years with Hank, whom she thought she would marry, but he eventually broke up with her. She was approaching forty and wanted to have a child, but there didn't seem to be anyone on the horizon that was a good prospect for a husband. She spent months talking about how she blamed Hank for misleading her. As she began to realize that blaming him was only adding to her depression, anger, and helplessness, we began to look at her situation from a problem-solving perspective.

Sharon was intelligent and resourceful, and she began to consider IVF. This was a major commitment, she felt, as a single woman, but she decided that trying to have a child was important enough for her. After many months of false starts and frustrations she finally got pregnant. She eventually left therapy, and a year later I got a card with a picture of Sharon holding her baby. She realized that blaming someone was less effective than solving her problem.

When we are blaming other people, our underlying belief is that we are helpless. But you are not helpless if you can solve a problem that is important to you.

Becoming a Victim

Many of the emotional difficulties we have arise from feeling like a victim. If you have been abused psychologically, physically, sexually, or in any other way, you truly have been a victim. We live in a world where even the people who claim they love us can treat us terribly. People can betray our trust. We can feel bewildered when someone we relied on was so malicious, treacherous, or unfeeling. There is no question that many of us have had experiences that leave us feeling disillusioned, distrustful, or resentful.

The question is not whether you have been a victim at some point. The question is: Are you defining your life as being a victim? Or are you more than a victim? Yes, your first response is to notice how hurt you feel, how unfair it has been, and how this has made your life worse. But if we get stuck on thinking of our identity as a victim, we render ourselves helpless.

One helpful response to feeling like a victim is to assert yourself, stand up for your rights, protest, seek restitution, seek redress, or get an apology. This may be the first useful response that you might take if someone mistreats you. It gives you a sense that you are willing to stand up for yourself, it is a way of exercising self-respect and self-esteem. *Assertion* is an important part of self-healing, and it requires recognizing that you are telling the other person how their behavior affected you, requesting a change, and telling them you are setting limits.

For example, Carolina told her friend Lisa that her critical comments were hurtful and that she wanted them to stop. And she added, "This is something we have talked about before. I want to keep you as a friend, but I also need to tell you that if you continue with your criticism, I will feel uncomfortable seeing you. I really want you to change this behavior toward me." Look at what was involved here. Carolina specified the behavior (critical comments), how it made her feel (hurt), and how she wanted her to change ("Stop criticizing me"). What she didn't do was label Lisa ("You're a terrible person"), escalate ("I will make you miserable if you do this again"), or completely discount their relationship (she said, "I want to keep you as a friend").

Assertion can sometimes work—sometimes the other person will change. But often it doesn't work, and you are left stating what your feelings are while the other person hasn't changed. This is when you have another choice.

Wendy's Story

Wendy was feeling stuck. Her former husband, Doug, had broken off their marriage and had filed for divorce. He had a history of being dismissive and critical of her feelings, telling her she was neurotic and that nothing could satisfy her. Wendy couldn't recall a single example of when he had validated her, told her he understood her feelings, or told her that her feelings made sense. He was the master at invalidation, and now he had left and didn't want to speak with her. She was on her own. Understandably, Wendy felt terrible. She felt betrayed, once again invalidated, humiliated, anxious. And she felt angry.

Two years later, she was still ruminating about the divorce, how he treated her, and how completely unfair it all was. Her anger and depression often kept her isolated from other people, because she felt that no one could really support her, no one wanted to hear about how terrible Doug had been, no one would make her feel better. She felt entitled to her anger. After all, he had criticized her once again, humiliated her, and then abandoned her. And, she was right. He had done those things. But now she was feeling stuck with her anger toward Doug, her resentments, and her loneliness. It was all his fault, she said, and there was nothing that she could do to change what happened two years ago.

Does Wendy have a right to feel upset? Yes, of course. Everyone has a right to any feeling they have, especially if treated unfairly. We can validate that. But ask yourself the following questions:

How long do you want to stay upset?

Will focusing repeatedly on the unfairness make your life better?

Is it possible to focus on positive goals to build your life while acknowledging that you were treated unfairly?

Even if you have a right to feeling upset, you also have a right to pursue other feelings, other goals, and other opportunities. You can acknowledge to yourself, "Yes, that wasn't fair and it shouldn't have happened, but now I am taking charge of my life." This doesn't invalidate the unfairness or the injury, but it does allow you to build your life and heal your wounds.

Repeatedly focusing on the injury may feel natural to you, and it may feel difficult to break away from that focus, but it also anchors you to the injury and keeps you from making your life better. If you rebuild your life and pursue positive goals, you may eventually care less about what happened in the past because you are now exercising more control over your life.

Sometimes we get caught up in the *victim identity trap*. We think of ourselves primarily as a victim. We may be right that we were treated badly, that this shouldn't have happened, but then we are hijacked by the identity of victim—and nothing else. When I have led workshops with therapists, I ask people to raise their hand if they have ever been treated unfairly. Almost everyone does so. Then I ask people if anyone close to them has broken their trust, betrayed them, or disappointed them in a serious way. Again, almost all hands go up. Including mine.

What can we make of this?

Life can be unfair, unpleasant, and unkind. But even when we are truly a victim, we are much more than the injury or hurt that we have suffered. We can validate the pain and the unfairness but still focus on what we can do to make our lives better.

Take-Home Points

◆ Your strategies for coping with uncomfortable emotions may be a bigger problem than the emotions themselves.

◆ Unhelpful coping strategies may escalate your negative feelings in the long term.

◆ Make it a goal to feel better for the long term, not the short term.

◆ Alcohol and drugs may calm emotions momentarily but will make everything worse.

◆ Binge eating will suppress emotions for a moment, but they will bounce back and be worse.

◆ Complaining may give some support but may alienate your friends.

◆ Reassurance seeking is normal, but it depends how you seek help.

◆ Avoiding uncomfortable situations reinforces your fear of feeling and limits your life.

◆ Blaming other people may have a grain of truth, but fixing the blame won't fix your problem.

◆ Ruminating and worrying will not give you the answer, and it will make you more depressed in the long term.

◆ It may be true that you have been treated unfairly, but getting stuck in the victim role is going to make you feel worse.

CHAPTER 11

Understanding How Other People Feel

Sometimes we are so caught up with our own thoughts and feelings that we say and do things without thinking about how others might experience us. We often fail to recognize what is going on in the hearts and minds of other people. It's also easy to misread someone else. In fact, sometimes we don't even recognize that the person before us is quite different from us at the current moment, that they have their own vulnerabilities, injuries, and needs. How can we connect better with the feelings of others?

Jenny likes to have a few drinks when she socializes, and she usually can be upbeat to be around. But when she is feeling high, she often will go off on negative tangents and become argumentative. When I asked Jenny how her friends experience her, she says, "Oh, my friends can be critical at times, but, you know, I am just trying to be myself."

Tom is another person whose emotions and self-absorption get in the way with people he cares about. When he talks with Luke, Tom just goes on about himself and doesn't ask Luke about what is going on with him. He is then surprised when Luke becomes angry at him and tells him that he is only interested in himself.

And then there's Jeff, who's been married for twenty-three years and came to see me because his wife threatened him with divorce. As Jeff described his interactions with his wife, it became clear that he yelled at her, criticized her, and humiliated her. I asked him, "Jeff, how do you think your wife feels about the way you handle her emotions?"

"I have no idea what you are talking about," was his response.

It's Not What You Say, It's What They Hear

We frequently don't pay attention to the impact we have on other people. We often get caught up in our own experience—our thoughts and feelings—and say things that we don't intend to be hurtful. After a while, we discover that we have alienated the very people we thought we could count on. And this is especially true when our friends and family members are going through a tough time. We may *intend* to be supportive, but we may end up making them feel misunderstood, uncared for, even criticized. Even if that was not our *intention*.

But in real life it's not what we say—it's what they hear. You may have the best intentions in talking to someone—you may sincerely want them to feel better—but what matters is what they hear, what your words mean to them. It's all about how they experience you.

Think about three people you see on a regular basis. Let's take your partner (if you have one, or a former partner), a close friend, and a family member. How do they experience you? When they are going through a tough time, do they feel comfortable opening up to you? Do you empathize with them or judge them? Do they think that you are going to be focused primarily on yourself? Take a few minutes to think this through and reflect on how this may affect your friendships and intimate relationships.

Just as your feelings are important to you, other people believe that their feelings are as important to them— and they may sometimes think that you don't understand them, care about them, or respect them. We are all a little *egocentric*—that is, we are caught up in our own perspective.

When a friend says something that I don't agree with, I automatically am captured by, caught up in, and sometimes hijacked by my own thoughts and feelings. I may want to tell them what I think, tell them they are wrong, even throw in a little sarcasm for good measure. But I have learned that this kind of banter only makes things worse and that things can escalate beyond control. And both of us will regret it. Just as my feelings are important to me, my friend's feelings are important to them. And, therefore, their feelings are important to me.

How Do People Respond to Your Feelings?

Before we examine your impact on others, let's start with understanding how it feels when others respond to your feelings. In the following exercise, we're going to look at negative responses in close relationships. Think about how a loved one responds to your feelings when you are upset. In the first column, read the different examples of how your loved one may respond when you are upset. In the second column, rate how true the responses are using the scale below. Then, in the third column, write out how their responses make you think and feel.

How My Loved One Responds to My Feelings

Scale:

    1 = Very untrue

    2 = Somewhat untrue

    3 = Slightly untrue

    4 = Slightly true

    5 = Somewhat true

    6 = Very true

How My Loved One Responds When I Am Upset	How True Is This? (1–6)	What Does Their Response Make Me Feel and Think?
Comprehensibility My loved one helps me make sense of my emotions.		
Validation My loved one helps me feel understood and cared for when I talk about my feelings.		
Guilt and shame My loved one criticizes me and tries to make me feel ashamed and guilty about the way I feel.		
Differentiation My loved one helps me understand that it is okay to have mixed feelings.		

How My Loved One Responds When I Am Upset	How True Is This? (1–6)	What Does Their Response Make Me Feel and Think?
Values My loved one relates my painful feelings to important values.		
Control My loved one thinks that I am out of control with my feelings.		
Numbness My loved one seems to be numb and indifferent when I talk about my feelings.		
Rational My loved one thinks I am irrational a lot of the time.		
Duration My loved one thinks that my painful feelings just go on and on.		
Consensus My loved one helps me realize that many people also feel the way I do.		
Acceptance My loved one accepts and tolerates my painful feelings and doesn't try to force me to change.		

How My Loved One Responds When I Am Upset	How True Is This? (1–6)	What Does Their Response Make Me Feel and Think?
Rumination My loved one seems to dwell on why I feel the way I feel.		
Expression My loved one encourages me to express my feelings and talk about the way I feel.		
Blame My loved one blames me for feeling so upset.		

Now, look back at these fourteen statements and consider the categories that ranked highest and lowest.

What are the three worst ways that your partner responds to you?

_____

_____

_____

What are the three best responses that your partner gives you?

_____

_____

_____

Allison and Ted's Story

Allison had been going through a lot of anxiety: panic attacks, fears of making mistakes, and worries about her health. She noted that Ted, her husband, would tell her that her feelings didn't make sense. He blamed her for her feelings, told her she was irrational, and complained that her feelings seemed to go on indefinitely. He also made her feel ashamed about her feelings, told her other people wouldn't feel this way, and labeled her feelings as out of control. Allison told me that these comments by Ted made her feel anxious, ashamed, angry, depressed, helpless, hopeless, and afraid of sharing her feelings with Ted. And Allison got more upset.

When I spoke with Ted, he agreed that Allison was often anxious and felt depressed. He added, "I do care about her, but she gets caught up in this continual emotional turmoil. I just want her to stop feeling bad." Ted had good intentions, he thought, but the impact on Allison only made things worse.

I asked Ted what he thought when Allison talked about her painful feelings. "I know she feels bad," he said, "but I think if she starts talking about how bad she feels she will just go on and on. She won't stop. It's too much for me at times. I try to get her to see things more positively, I try to get her to calm down, but then she tells me that I don't understand. I don't know what to do with her. I want her to stop feeling bad."

Ted has certain beliefs about Allison's emotions:

I want her to stop feeling bad.

I can't stand it when she is upset.

Once she starts talking about her emotions, she won't stop complaining about how she feels.

I have to get her to stop feeling bad right now.

She won't listen to me. If she did, she would feel better.

Talking about feelings often makes things worse.

She is too emotional.

She is neurotic.

Ted has several theories about Allison's feelings. He believes, "Her emotions don't make sense and therefore she shouldn't have these feelings. Painful emotions are bad, and I have to get her to stop feeling that way. If I don't get her to stop feeling bad, she will get worse and go on complaining indefinitely. Her emotions are a burden to me, and at the same time I feel responsible for getting her to feel better. If she doesn't change the way she feels when I tell her that her feelings don't make any sense, then she doesn't respect me. If I indulge her and try to validate her, I will be reinforcing her complaining and things will get worse. She will overwhelm me with her emotions."

Ted's beliefs about Allison's feelings reflect his negative beliefs about emotions. He views her emotions as partly his responsibility to control, and if she doesn't "listen" to him (obey), then she doesn't really want to change her feelings and is being disrespectful. I asked Ted what he was concerned about.

He said, "Look, if I just talk to her about her feelings, then there will be no place for my feelings. She doesn't realize how hard I work to support the family, she just complains about everything. I never get any appreciation. She takes me for granted. You know, I would like some validation too."

"How did your parents respond to you, Ted, when you were a kid—when you were upset?" I asked.

"My father always wanted me to be perfect. He only wanted me to talk about my success. Just last week I was talking with him about my work and he asked me how things were going . I said, 'Things are going well,' and he said, 'That's what I want to hear. Things are going well. That's what I expect from you.'"

I said, "How does that make you feel that he only wants to hear about your good experiences, your positive feelings?"

"It makes me think he doesn't care about me. I never got any validation from him. He never understood me."

How ironic that Ted, who never felt validated, seldom validates Allison? He learned from a young age—primarily from his father—that feelings were a burden, the other person had to get rid of those feelings, and getting validated would never happen. Ted was copying his father's invalidating approach and found it hard to accept Allison's feelings.

Your Beliefs About the Emotions of Other People

All of us have a theory about the emotions of other people. This theory—based on the *emotional schema model*—includes our beliefs about how long someone's emotions should last, whether they are legitimate, whether they are out of control, and whether they are different from those of other people. We also have our own theories or strategies about how to respond to the emotions of other people. This includes many negative responses such as:

- Minimizing their experience: "It's not that important."

- Toxic positivity: "It will all work out."

- Criticism: "You are being a big baby about this."

- Suppression: "Get a hold of yourself."

- Blaming the past: "You are like this because of your crazy family."

- Stonewalling: refusing to listen

- Avoiding: walking out of the room

- Ridiculing: "Look at you—such a child. What's wrong with you?"

- Personalizing: "Don't blame me for your problems."

- Problem solving: "I can tell you how to solve this problem."

- Overcontrol of the situation: "I will take care of this."

Every time that we interact with people, we are dealing with their emotions. You may think that your partner's emotions annoy you, overwhelm you, or that they are a burden to you. Or you may think that your friend's emotions seem to go on forever, don't make sense, or are a sign of their self-absorption. But as much as you may feel affected by their emotions, the fact is that we never really see these emotions. We only see what they do, what they say, and how they interact with us. We have a hard time knowing what is going on inside the other person.

Mutual Misunderstandings

Brenda thinks that Ken is irritated with her. She asks him, "Why are you talking to me that way?" Which surprises him because he has said very little to her. He is trying to read her mind, and he comes up with the idea that she doesn't like his driving. She hasn't said anything about his driving, but that is his theory for the moment about her irritability with him.

Now notice the leaps of belief for Ken: Brenda is irritated with him, and she doesn't like his driving. He could be right, but he doesn't really know. Right now Ken is stuck in his mind reading about Brenda. He doesn't know the range of emotions that she is experiencing, and he doesn't know why she feels what she is feeling. He is also taking it personally—that she is feeling whatever she is feeling because she is angry with him. He doesn't realize that her feelings may be about something else.

He then continues thinking about her emotions. Ken's stream of consciousness begins to unravel: "She is going to go on forever with this mood" (duration), "Her feelings don't make sense" (lack of comprehensibility), "She is going to get worse and worse" (lack of control, escalation), "She shouldn't feel this way" (blaming), "I have to get her to stop feeling this way" (need for control), "I can't accept this" (lack of acceptance), and "Why can't she be more rational and reasonable?" (anti-emotional rationality).

As a result of these negative interpretations of Brenda's emotions, Ken becomes defensive: "Leave me alone, I'm driving." He starts to distance himself from Brenda, not wanting to talk to her. He thinks, "If we continue talking, she is going to get more irritable and start nitpicking. Better for me to keep quiet." He stops talking to her and begins to ruminate about her emotions. He thinks, "This has been going on for years. She is so moody. I don't know what the hell she wants from me." Ken has reached the point that he cannot accept whatever emotions Brenda is experiencing. He thinks she has to stop feeling this way, and he thinks that he has to get her to stop.

As Ken becomes more distant—and, at the same time, more irritated with Brenda—Brenda begins thinking that Ken is moody, irritable, and doesn't communicate. At first she wonders what she has done to elicit this kind of moodiness, and she can't see what is making him so annoyed. She then begins thinking about his emotions: "Ken is moody and irritable. He is always like this" (over-generalizing), "This is going to go on for the entire day" (duration), "He can get really irritable and angry" (escalation), "I have to get him to stop feeling this way" (low acceptance), "He has no control over his feelings" (lack of control), "His feelings don't make any sense" (incomprehensible).

Does any of this sound familiar?

All of us are engaged in mind reading about the emotions of other people. Sometimes we are correct and sometimes we aren't. But we make guesses about the feelings of the people in our lives, and we have our explanations and evaluations of these feelings. Let's look again at what was actually going on with Ken and Brenda.

It turns out that Ken was feeling upset that Brenda was going away on a business trip in another week. She was going to be gone for two weeks, and he was going to miss her. He was feeling sad about this, and he was anxious about being alone without her. Ken knew he would miss her. Although he knew she had every right to pursue her professional career, he felt personally rejected. He wished that she wouldn't travel as much as she did. Ken felt that a "real man" shouldn't be so dependent on his wife—shouldn't be so needy. So, he was trying to act like he didn't need her although he knew he really did. So, Ken had a wide range of his own emotions—anxious and sad about Brenda being away, and angry that he felt this way while blaming her for his feelings of dependency, and then feeling ashamed of his own feelings.

How about Brenda? She was also feeling anxious about her business trip and even more anxious that Ken was going on his own business trip a few days after she was going to return. They would be apart from each other for three of the next five weeks, and they felt really connected to each other. But this connection made Brenda anxious. She would miss him while she was away and miss him even more when he was away. So she was feeling anxious and sad too. (Sounds a lot like Ken, doesn't it?) Because she was anxious about their respective independent trips, she was especially sensitive to any tone in Ken's voice. She frequently felt anxious when he traveled, and she often felt that Ken was rejecting her when he was irritable. Brenda didn't want to have a bad time before she left on her trip.

What is ironic about their experiences is that neither one had a clue as to what was going on inside the other person. They were partially correct that the other person felt irritated, but they didn't realize the range of emotions that the other person felt. And they were off the mark in understanding why the other person was feeling what they were feeling.

We typically explain another person's emotions by referring to a *stable trait* or quality that they have: "She is moody" or "He is irritable." It's as if we think that their moods never change, that they are always moody or irritable. We don't recognize how variable their emotions may be. We tend to attribute their emotions to "something about them" rather than something about the situation or something about the way we affect them at the present moment. This is partly because we also have difficulty understanding how our behavior impacts the other person (egocentric bias).

We look at the other person and we see them as a "whole person"—that is, we are visually focused on what they sound like and look like right now. We don't recognize how complex and variable other people may be, because we are looking at them as "one person" rather than thinking about how their behavior and moods fluctuate over time and situations.

We don't take their visual perspective and see ourselves from their eyes. We are caught in our own perspective, unable to see the world from their perspective, unable to see how they change, unable to recognize what we don't know about them. As a result we label them: moody, irritable, neurotic.

How to Be More Supportive and Effective

Ken, Brenda, and I looked at the different interpretations of what happened. As they began to realize that they had misinterpreted the emotions of their partner, they began to feel relieved. In fact, their irritability was a sign of their connectedness.

Ken examined his interpretations of Brenda's emotions.

Ken's Initial Interpretation of Brenda's Emotions	Type of Thought	More Helpful View of Brenda's Emotions
She is going to go on forever with this mood.	Duration	No, Brenda's feelings are just like mine—they change over time. She was in a good mood a little while ago, and she is likely to be in a good mood later.
Her feelings don't make sense.	Lack of comprehensibility	They may make sense if I knew what she was thinking and feeling. But I don't. Perhaps she has something on her mind. Perhaps she is anxious about being away and my being away.
She is going to get worse and worse.	Lack of control, escalation	That doesn't always seem to be the case. I have noticed that her feelings change depending on what we are doing or to whom she is speaking.
She shouldn't feel this way.	Blaming	It's not helpful for me to judge her feelings. There is nothing immoral about having an emotion. She is not harming anyone with her feelings. People have a right to their feelings.
I have to get her to stop feeling this way.	Need for control	No, I don't have to get her to stop feeling this way. I can validate her, encourage her to express how she feels, understand where she is coming from. I can allow her to be herself and love her.

I can't accept this.	Lack of acceptance	Why can't I accept her feelings? She is having her feelings right now, and there is no sense in not accepting them. Her feelings are her feelings for the present moment.
Why can't she be more rational and reasonable?	Overly rational	Maybe she is being rational and reasonable from her point of view. Maybe I don't know what she is thinking and feeling right now. I can ask her and be patient and not argue with her. By the way—it's not rational to expect people to always be rational. Humans are not wired that way.

Let's go back to the worksheet "How My Loved One Responds to My Feelings." You may recall that each of the negative responses and beliefs that your partner has about your emotions (for example, that your feelings don't make sense, that you do not need to be validated, that other people don't feel the way you do) only makes you feel worse.

But now, let's look at how you think about the emotions that your loved one has. Do you have any of these beliefs about their emotions? In the first column, read the different examples of how you may respond to your loved one when they are upset. In the second column, rate how true the responses are using the scale below. Then, in the third column, write out how your responses make them think and feel.

How I Respond to My Partner's Emotions

Scale:

1 = Very untrue

2 = Somewhat untrue

3 = Slightly untrue

4 = Slightly true

5 = Somewhat true

6 = Very true

How I Respond to My Loved One's Feelings	How True Is This?	What Does This Make Them Feel and Think?
Comprehensibility I help my loved one make sense of their emotions.		
Validation I help them feel understood and cared for when they talk about their feelings.		
Guilt or shame I criticize them and make them feel ashamed and guilty about the way they feel.		
Differentiation I help them understand that it is okay to have mixed feelings.		

How I Respond to My Loved One's Feelings	How True Is This?	What Does This Make Them Feel and Think?
Values I relate their feelings to important values.		
Control I think that their feelings are out of control.		
Numbness I often feel numb and indifferent when they talk about their feelings.		
Rational I think that they are irrational a lot of the time.		
Duration I think that their painful feelings just go on and on.		
Consensus I realize that many people also feel the way they feel.		
Acceptance I accept and tolerate their painful feelings and don't try to force them to change.		

How I Respond to My Loved One's Feelings	How True Is This?	What Does This Make Them Feel and Think?
Rumination I think over and over and seem to dwell on why they feel what they feel.		
Expression I encourage them to express their feelings and talk about the way they feel.		
Blame I blame them for feeling so upset.		

Now, look back at these fourteen statements and consider the categories that ranked highest and lowest.

What are the three best responses that you give to your loved one?

_____

_____

_____

What are the three worst ways that you respond to your loved one?

_____

_____

_____

Now, imagine how you would feel if other people—especially someone close to you—responded to your painful feelings this way. You would be hurt, anxious, angry, misunderstood. You would think that there is no sense in sharing your feelings with this person. I'm willing to bet that this is not your intention when you are talking to someone that you love and care about. You probably want them to feel better, but your beliefs about emotion only get in the way. In fact, they make things worse.

Let's take a look at how you can challenge these beliefs about your loved one's painful emotions. In the following table, look for some common negative responses that you have. Then see what a more helpful response would be. You can also find helpful examples of positive responses (such as validation) that you'd like to use more often.

Examples of Helpful Responses to My Partner's Feelings

How I Respond to My Loved One's Feelings	Helpful Responses
Comprehensibility I help my loved one make sense of their emotions.	"Your feelings make sense given what you are going through. There are a lot of things that you are thinking right now and experiencing that lead you to feel this way."
Validation I help them feel understood and cared for when they talk about their feelings.	"Of course you feel upset, look at what you are going through. You have every right to feel the way that you feel. It must be hard for you, and I want you to know that I am here for you."
Guilt or shame I criticize them and make them feel ashamed and guilty about the way they feel.	"You are feeling the way you feel, and that is okay. You have every right to those feelings. You are human."
Differentiation I help them understand that it is okay to have mixed feelings	"There are a lot of times when we all have mixed feelings. That's because things are seldom as simple as we would like them to be. You have a richness of feelings—a wide range of emotions. We all do."
Values I relate their feelings to important values.	"Things bother you at times because you value certain things. These are things that are important to you, because you know there are important things in life. You care about these things."

How I Respond to My Loved One's Feelings	Helpful Responses
Control I think that their feelings are out of control.	"Your feelings go up and down, and they seem to take you on a roller coaster. But you have been on this ride before, and it eventually does slow down. Right now it feels like a rough and unsteady journey for you."
Numbness I often feel numb and indifferent when they talk about their feelings.	"I can feel some of the pain that you are feeling, and I know it must hurt you even more. I want you to know that I am feeling compassion and love for you during this time."
Rational I think that they are irrational a lot of the time.	"There is no need to be rational. We are not robots, we are not computers. We are human. Our emotions are real and important and tell us what matters to us."
Duration I think that their painful feelings just go on and on.	"I know it seems as if your painful feelings will last forever. But we've been here before, and let's hope together that the painful feelings will slow down, quiet down, and become less painful."
Consensus I realize that many people also feel the way they feel.	"You are not alone with these feelings. We all go through difficult times. You and I have had painful feelings and so have many other people, and many of these feelings are exactly what you are feeling right now. You are human and you are having the feelings that humans have when life is difficult."
Acceptance I accept and tolerate their painful feelings and don't try to force them to change.	"I am here with you and accept and hear what you are feeling. We can ride this out together. You will feel what you are feeling until those feelings change. But right now they are real, and we can make room for them, accept them, and maybe learn from them."
Rumination I think over and over and seem to dwell on why they feel the way they feel.	"I can see that you are feeling the way you are feeling. I know that this is tough for you, but I will be here. I know that you are having a hard time, and even if some things are hard to understand, they are still real. Your feelings are what is important right now."

How I Respond to My Loved One's Feelings	Helpful Responses
Expression I encourage them to express their feelings and talk about the way they feel.	*"You can tell me anything that you are feeling, and I will try to hear what you are saying, understand you, and support you. I am here for you, right here, right now."*
Blame I blame them for feeling so upset.	*"You have a right to your feelings. I would never blame you for having a headache or indigestion, and your feelings are part of your experience."*

Now that you have learned some helpful responses to say to your loved one when they are talking about their feelings, let's keep track of examples of you doing these things during the next week. Starting today, write out examples of your responses each day to someone's feelings using the worksheet that follows.

Helpful Responses to My Loved One's Feelings

How I Respond to My Loved One's Feelings	Name of Loved One	My Helpful Response
Comprehensibility I help my loved one make sense of their emotions.		
Validation I help them feel understood and cared for when they talk about their feelings.		
Guilt or shame I criticize them and make them feel ashamed and guilty about the way they feel.		
Differentiation I help them understand that it's okay to have mixed feelings.		
Values I relate their feelings to important values.		
Control I think that their feelings are out of control.		
Numbness I often feel numb and indifferent when they talk about their feelings.		

How I Respond to My Loved One's Feelings	Name of Loved One	My Helpful Response
Rational I think that they are irrational a lot of the time.		
Duration I think that their painful feelings just go on and on.		
Consensus I realize that many people also feel the way they feel.		
Acceptance I accept and tolerate their painful feelings and don't try to force them to change.		
Rumination I think over and over and seem to dwell on why they feel the way they feel.		
Expression I encourage them to express their feelings and talk about the way they feel.		
Blame I blame them for feeling so upset.		

Take-Home Points

+ Think about how it feels when a loved one does not support your emotional experience.

+ When a loved one is upset, notice how you respond to them.

+ Notice whether you sound critical or dismissive. Notice if you are minimizing their feelings or telling them that they shouldn't feel the way that they feel.

+ Even if your intentions are good, remember that it is what they are hearing—the impact on them—that matters. It's not what you say, it's what they hear.

+ Ask yourself how you can communicate respect, warmth, and acceptance of your loved one's feelings.

+ Using the emotional schema model, you can help your loved one feel that you believe their emotions make sense, that others have similar feelings, that you validate them, that their feelings are not out of control, and that having mixed feelings sometimes makes sense. You can encourage your loved one to express their feelings, link their feelings to important values, and help them feel less ashamed about their emotions.

CHAPTER 12

Putting It All Together: The Best Ways to Cope

We have covered a lot of territory in how to understand your emotions, use them productively, and not get hijacked by them. Now it's time to provide a summary of the many ideas and techniques that you can use so that you can have a better relationship with your emotions. Keep in mind that the goal of emotional schema therapy is not to get rid of your emotions—it is to be able to live with them, learn from them, and cope effectively with them.

In this chapter, you will learn eight steps that you can use with any emotion. Each of the steps has been discussed in detail in earlier chapters; here we bring them together.

1. Validate Your Feelings

One of the messages that we get about certain emotions is: *You are not supposed to feel that way.* You may have heard your parents, partner, or friends say that you shouldn't be upset, you shouldn't feel jealous, you shouldn't feel envious. Maybe someone told you that you have so much going for you that you shouldn't feel sad. These dismissive and invalidating comments are hurtful and only make you feel worse. And, in fact, you may even be saying these things to yourself, such as, "I don't have any right to feel this way." You may be invalidating yourself, and you feel bad about feeling bad.

We would never tell someone that they shouldn't have a headache. Why does it make sense to tell someone that they should never feel sad, anxious, angry, or hurt?

For instance, you may feel embarrassed about crying. But crying is part of human nature, and one of the worst things that can happen when you're struggling is to believe that no one cares about your crying. Perhaps you have been told, "Stop crying," which made you hold in the pain, hold back the tears, and feel alone in your suffering.

The emotional schema approach recognizes that painful feelings and crying are part of human existence. In fact, the saddest thing in life is to never have anything worth crying over. Validating your feelings can begin with acknowledging and supporting yourself when you feel down. You can say to yourself that you understand that life can be very difficult, that you feel overwhelmed, and that things may seem hopeless at times. You have a right to whatever feelings you have.

One way to validate your feelings is to *normalize* them—to universalize them. This means that we can recognize that people worldwide often have the same feelings. In fact, all of our emotions—especially our fears of heights, strangers, closed spaces, or being left alone—have evolved to protect us. Even complicated emotions like jealousy, envy, shame, and guilt have evolved because they protected us or assured social cohesiveness. And our current feelings are often related to the messages about what we should be like—the rules and regulations our parents laid down. Validating our feelings can include realizing that all of these factors have led to our current experience.

Your feelings are important. Telling yourself that you have a right to have feelings is the first step in validating yourself. You can also direct compassion and kindness toward yourself—just as you would with a loved one. You can comfort yourself by saying to yourself, "Although life is hard at the present moment, I will love myself, take care of myself, and support myself through this difficult time." You need to say to yourself, "I am here for me, I will take care of the feelings I have, listen to my pain, and help support myself to get to the next step." And that step can lead to feeling differently.

Feeling differently does not invalidate your pain. No, it tells you that you matter enough that changing that pain is an act of kindness to yourself.

2. Learn the Lessons of Emotional Schema Therapy

Yes, life is complicated, unfair, difficult, and feels impossible at times. But a full life includes all of those things—and the ability to *feel everything,* not just *feel good.* The emotional schema therapy approach to emotions—and indeed to a full life—includes the following principles:

- Difficult and unpleasant emotions are part of everyone's experience.

- Emotions warn us, tell us about our needs, and connect us with meaning.

- Beliefs about emotions can make it difficult for us to tolerate our feelings.

- Strategies for coping with our emotions can make matters better or worse.

Remember that *emotional realism,* as opposed to *emotional perfectionism,* implies that we need to be ready for the full range of emotions, that we will not always be happy, and that all of us will face disappointments, even disillusionment, at times. I refer to *existential perfectionism,* which means that our lives will not be exactly what we want them to be. It means that we will have friends who let us down, just as we let them down. It means that life involves tradeoffs, compromises, getting along with people we don't like. We can think of emotional perfectionism as a part of existential perfectionism. With emotional perfectionism, we want our emotions to be happy, good, and clear. With existential perfectionism we not only want those pleasant emotions all the time but we want all aspects of our lives to be good, to live up to our demanding and often unrealistic expectations. You also learned about *constructive discomfort,* which means that to make progress we have to do things that are uncomfortable. It means that we build resilience and even mental toughness by valuing the ability to tolerate difficult experiences and overcome obstacles. You want to be able to say to yourself, "I am the person who does the hard things."

One valuable way of empowering yourself is to realize that your goal is to *do what you don't want to do.* This involves the ability to overcome inertia, feeling stuck, and waiting for your motivation to show up.

It means that it will be up to you to take your life back.

3. Recognize That Emotions Are Temporary

Our emotions often mislead us into thinking that they will go on forever—or at least a very long time. But even feelings like hopelessness are temporary. How do we know? Because by keeping track of our emotions every hour of the week—as you did in the exercise "How Long Will This Feeling Last" in chapter 5—we find that the intensity of our emotions changes with what we are doing, who we are with, what we are thinking, and even with the time of day. Emotions change, and knowing this should give us hope. *This, too, will pass.*

If we believe that our emotions are permanent, we will avoid situations that activate uncomfortable feelings. This avoidance further reinforces our negative beliefs about emotions and keeps us from living a full life. Our belief about the permanence of emotion also leads us to believe that we are our emotions. For example, you might think, "I am a depressed person," rather than thinking, "In certain situations and at certain times I feel depressed to various degrees."

There is no such thing as a "depressed person." There are people who experience depression at times, under certain circumstances. Your eye color won't change, but your depression will.

We also tend to predict that if something negative happens in the future, our emotions will last indefinitely. This is the illusion of the durability of emotion and seems to be part of human nature, because we all do this at times. Our beliefs about emotion are often exaggerated—if not plain wrong. The fact is, there are many factors that will affect the variability of our emotions in the future. For example, if we believe that if we have a breakup or lose something of value then we will be unhappy forever, we will dread the future and worry about terrible things happening. But our predictions about our future emotions often ignore the experiences that can help us cope with difficulties. For example, we tend to focus on our current emotion to predict our future emotions, rather than recognizing that new friends, new relationships, a new job, and new experiences may give rise to different and happier feelings.

The other factor that affects how we think about our current negative emotions is that we don't recall how our past negative feelings came to an end. This is because when we are unhappy we tend to over-recall negative past events and feelings, and not recall positive experiences—our memory is biased by our current emotions. It is like viewing the world through dark glasses and concluding that night will go on forever. We can take the glasses off and see that we have a wide range of positive and negative emotions.

Emotions are temporary—although they may fool us into thinking that they will last forever.

4. Feel Less Guilty and Ashamed About Your Feelings

A lot of us have heard our parents or partners tell us that we shouldn't feel the way we do. We have heard, "You shouldn't feel jealous" or "You should appreciate what you have—you should not be depressed." We have heard that we are weak, childish, neurotic, or simply crazy and stupid because we have the feelings we have. Perhaps someone bullied you when you were a kid, perhaps you have been humiliated because of your feelings. This humiliation can focus on your sexual desires, your fears, or your worries about the future. You have been made to feel bad about feeling what you feel.

But feelings don't hurt other people—it's only actions that hurt. And your emotions—fear, anger, jealousy, hopelessness—are part of your experience. You may also feel guilty about an emotion—or a fantasy—because you think that it is dangerous, that it is a sign that something bad will happen. But feelings are not the same thing as choices. You can feel angry without acting in a hostile way. You can have sexual fantasies without acting on them. Your feelings of guilt or shame may have come from someone who misunderstood you, who doesn't really understand emotion or human nature. Why hand over your self-esteem to someone who doesn't understand?

They may label you irrational, neurotic, or crazy. But every emotion that you have—every fantasy—is the same as those of millions, if not billions, of people. We are all feeling the same things. But our emotions are harmless—they are not the same as actions.

Just as no one is harmed by your indigestion, no one is harmed by the feelings inside of you.

5. Make Room for Your Emotions

You may think that your goal is to get rid of any negative feelings, but if you are going to live a complete life you will have a full range of feelings—some wonderful, some happy, some sad, and some, at times, really awful. I know I have. And I suspect that in the future I will have that full range again—even the awful. We often have beliefs in emotional perfectionism—that our minds should be clear, our emotions should make us feel good all the time, that happiness is the goal every day. But then we learn that this quest for the Holy Grail of Happy Feelings is a mirage. It's not happening—it won't happen.

If we realize that our goal is to be okay with feeling everything, then we can make room for the emotions that come. You learned a wide range of techniques to help with accepting your emotions, including *thinking of the bigger picture* in your life, that is, that there are many experiences and many possibilities that you have faced and will face, both positive and negative. This helps you see the larger context, the wider scope. There is plenty of room, along with all the other emotions, for the emotion you are having right now.

We can think about our emotions as residing in a large lake of feelings, with new feelings—some negative—as streams that empty into the larger lake. There is room here for those feelings.

We can also think about our emotions as a balloon that pulls us in one direction and then in another. But if we choose, we can let go of the string and let the balloon drift away. We can let our feelings go.

And we can imagine our emotions as jabbering away, like a talking silly clown that keeps warning us that life is a disaster. But we can allow the clown to have that silly voice and still get on with doing what we need to do to make our lives meaningful. We don't have to be controlled by a clown.

We can feel more in control of our feelings if we temporarily let go of a goal that is attached to those feelings and focus on another goal. For example, I woke this morning a little frustrated about some professional goals, but I decided to work on this chapter and, to be honest with you, I have gotten my mind off of the goal that made me frustrated.

Sometimes giving up is getting on. If we change our goals, our feelings may change in a different direction.

We can even make an appointment with our emotions. For example, if you are jealous, you can make an appointment with your jealousy, or if you are angry you can make an appointment with your anger, as you did similarly in the exercise "Using Worry Time." Putting off your uncomfortable emotion until later may sound difficult, if not impossible. But it is possible. Ask yourself, "What am I telling myself that is making this so important? Is this really worth getting this angry about? How will I feel about this a week from now, a month from now, a year from now?" Stepping away and questioning your emotion may be the first step in letting it go.

6. Learn to Live with Your Ambivalence

There are times when we think that we should feel only one way. We may think that mixed feelings are a bad sign, that we cannot make a decision if we are ambivalent. This is part of our emotional perfectionism—looking for the maximum, the best, or absolute certainty. But mixed feelings are part of life.

You will have mixed feelings about your best friend, and they will have mixed feelings about you. The same can be true with your partner—mutual ambivalence. You will have mixed feelings about your work, where you live, your desires for someone, even your next meal. Mixed feelings don't mean something is wrong; they mean that you are being open and honest about the pros and cons of experiences in your life. That's because life is not black and white. It's more like a kaleidoscope that continually changes, continually clashes. Life is full of noise.

Life is complex—and it is constantly changing. Every choice involves tradeoffs, upsides, and downsides. There is no choice that you couldn't question at another time. We often get hijacked and misled trying to seek closure, certainty, and clarity, but life involves conflict, confusion, and change. It's like a symphony that is rewritten on a daily basis—the melody sounds somewhat familiar but the notes are changing. Even the players are changing.

We can give up on *pure mind*—the belief in black-and-white thinking—and recognize that nothing is so clear and simple, because we never have all the information and everything involves tradeoffs. Certain things come with the territory. There is no free lunch.

Searching for certainty and clarity may only lead to rumination and constant questioning. Why do you need clarity and certainty? Why keep asking yourself, "How do I really feel?" Maybe the way you really feel is ambivalent.

And that is okay.

Maybe ambivalence is part of emotional realism—living in the real world of complexity, fluidity, and openness. Rather than look at ambivalence as a problem, you can look at it as a realistic view of how you feel—that is, as part of your full range of emotions.

A symphony requires many notes and several movements. Notes and movements complement and enrich the final piece of music. Maybe our feelings are like that.

7. Clarify Your Values

Our emotions are often connected to our values or what we think at the moment is important. But sometimes we find ourselves losing sight of the bigger picture of our lives, of what truly matters, and we get upset about distractions and disruptions that are more an inconvenience than a central issue in our lives. If you have suffered a real loss or injury—the death of someone you cared about or abuse and harassment by someone in authority—then you know what really matters. But we often get distracted being upset about what someone else thinks, or by feeling misunderstood, or by not having things our way. Our emotions get carried away. This is especially true when it comes to anger.

There are many ways of determining what your core values are. One way is to imagine your own funeral and ask yourself what you would want people to say about you. What would you want to have your life mean for others? What would be the highlights of your life? If you can identify the kind of person you would want to be remembered as, then try to become that person.

Another technique that can help you is using *negation*. You can imagine that everything you are and have has been taken away. The only way you can get anything back is to ask for it one at a time—and make a case for your appreciation of it. So often the things and experiences that we would miss and desperately want back are often right in front of us. But we need to open our eyes to see.

Think about the qualities of someone you admire. Perhaps they are kindness, generosity, self-discipline, intelligence, reliability, flexibility, forgiveness, acceptance, or courage. Then, each day engage in behavior that reflects the qualities.

When we live according to our values, we still will feel upset about things—but we can also view our experience as having the right feelings about the right things. For example, it makes sense to be upset about learning that someone you know has been abused. Your empathy and compassion for the other person connects you with your values. Your emotions at times can be painful, but for the right reasons.

Sometimes when you are honest with yourself, certain people won't like you. Unfortunately, that is the price you may have to pay. It simply means that they cannot accept what reality is—that people disagree with each other. That is their problem, not yours.

8. Understand the Emotions of Other People

All of us are prone to getting caught up in our own perspective and misunderstanding of the emotions of other people. Think about how difficult it is to really understand what someone else is thinking and feeling. This is a fundamental dilemma in human existence and gives rise to misunderstandings, failure to empathize, and conflicts that are usually in the imaginations of people who really care for each other. This is particularly true in intimate relationships and close friendships.

Each of us has a theory about the emotions of other people. For example, when a loved one is upset, you may believe that they are always upset, that they will go on and on, that their feelings don't make sense, and that they shouldn't feel the way they do. This can lead you to invalidate them, dismiss their feelings, or try to control them by getting them to change the way that they feel. That usually backfires.

So, think about how you respond to their feelings and ask yourself, "When I am upset, how do I want my loved ones to respond to me?" Very likely you would want them to take time to listen, validate you, not judge you, and help you understand that your feelings make sense and that others would feel the same way.

Keep in mind that when you respond to others you may be well intentioned, but the impact on the other person might backfire. For example, you might offer advice, but your offer may be viewed as patronizing and invalidating. This is the difference between intention and impact. It's not what you say, it's what they hear. What do you want them to hear?

Make room for the feelings and thoughts of others. Know that you don't have to agree with them; simply respect their experience. We often think that people close to us should see things exactly the way we do. But we are different and, indeed, our own thoughts and feelings change—so why should our loved ones be a copy of who we are?

If I asked your loved one how you respond to their feelings, would they be pleased? Would they be disappointed? Would they feel criticized for their feelings? What would you like them to say?

Final Thoughts

We are all human and, as such, we need to learn to live with the full range of emotions that have evolved to warn us, protect us, and connect us. Sometimes our emotional messages lead us astray—to believe that our emotions will last forever, escalate to catastrophic levels, or confuse us.

We have learned that certain emotions are not okay, that we are wrong, guilty, or shameful to have these emotions. But our strong emotions are an inevitable part of human existence. We would not condemn someone for having allergies, or for feeling tired or hungry.

Recognizing our emotions and listening to them, keeping in mind our goals and what we value, and imagining the advice of our future self is the beginning of wisdom. It is up to each of us to find the path, along with our feelings, that will lead us to where we want to go.

Acknowledgments

I want to start by thanking Matthew McKay, the publisher of New Harbinger Publications, who suggested that I write this book based on his interest in the emotional schema model. It also helped that Matthew laughed at my jokes over lunch, which suggested that his insights should be taken seriously. I want to thank my editor, Ryan Buresh, who has been supportive of the work I have done with him and for his openness about changes in the structure of this work. The editorial staff at New Harbinger has been diligent and helpful at every step along the way. My thanks to Marisa Solís, Caleb Beckwith, and Clancy Drake for their careful editing as the book unfolded.

I am especially grateful, once again, to my masterful literary agent, Bob Diforio, who has been part of my journey for many years and has guided me with his skill and wisdom.

Writing a book is a group effort, and this book reflects the many contributions of my colleagues worldwide whose work has influenced my thinking. I want to thank Aaron Beck, David A. Clark, Paul Gilbert, Steve Hayes, Stefan Hofmann, Marsha Linehan, John Riskind, and Adrian Wells, whose creative insights into helping people overcome suffering have inspired me and many others. I also want to thank my colleagues at the American Institute for Cognitive Therapy in New York City (www.CognitiveTherapyNYC.com) who have been patient and warmly critical in helping me develop these ideas. Our weekly case conferences have made this and many other projects possible. My research assistant, Nicolette Molina, has been a dedicated support throughout every phase of this project.

And much of my understanding about life and emotion is owed to my wife, Helen, who always has an insight about something to which I may often be blind. It is to her that this book is gratefully dedicated.

References

Chapter 2

Appel, H., A. L. Gerlach, and J. Crusius. 2016. "The Interplay Between Facebook Use, Social Comparison, Envy, and Depression." *Current Opinion in Psychology* 9: 44–49.

Bornstein, M. H., D. L. Putnick, P. Rigo, G. Esposito, J. E. Swain, J. T. D. Suwalsky, et al. 2017. "Neurobiology of Culturally Common Maternal Responses to Infant Cry." *Proceedings of the National Academy of Sciences* 114(45): E9465–E9473. https://doi.org/10.1073/pnas.1712022114.

De Pisapia, N., M. H. Bornstein, P. Rigo, G. Esposito, S. De Falco, and P. Venuti. 2013. "Gender Differences in Directional Brain Responses to Infant Hunger Cries." *Neuroreport* 24(3)" 142.

Ehrenreich, S. E., and M. K. Underwood. 2016. "Adolescents' Internalizing Symptoms as Predictors of the Content of their Facebook Communication and Responses Received from Peers." *Translational Issues in Psychological Science* 2(3): 227.

Gilbert, P. 2009. *The Compassionate Mind*. London: Constable.

Kessler, R. C., P. Berglund, O. Demler, R. Jin, K. R., Merikangas, and E. E. Walters. 2005. "Lifetime Prevalence and Age-of-Onset Distributions of DSM-IV Disorders in the National Comorbidity Survey Replication." *Archives of General Psychiatry* 62(6): 593–602.

Lingle, S., M. T. Wyman, R. Kotrba, L. J. Teichroeb, and C. A. Romanow. 2012. "What Makes a Cry a Cry? A Review of Infant Distress Vocalizations." *Current Zoology* 58(5): 698–726.

Chapter 4

Leahy, R. L. 2015. *Emotional Schema Therapy*. New York: Guilford Publications.

Leahy, R. L. 2018. "Emotional Schema Therapy: A Social-Cognitive Model." In R. L. Leahy (Ed.) *Science and Practice in Cognitive Therapy: Foundations, Mechanisms, and Applications*. New York: Guilford.

Miller, S. 2004. *Gilgamesh: A New English Version*. New York: The Free Press.

Chapter 5

Dweck, C. S. 2006. *Mindset: The New Psychology of Success*. New York: Random House.

Gilbert, P. 1998. "The Evolved Basis and Adaptive Functions of Cognitive Distortions." *British Journal of Medical Psychology* 71: 447–463.

Leahy, R. L., D. D. Tirch, and P. S. Melwani. 2012. "Processes Underlying Depression: Risk Aversion, Emotional Schemas, and Psychological Flexibility." *International Journal of Cognitive Therapy* 5(4): 362–379.

Lyubomirsky, S. 2011. "Hedonic Adaptation to Positive and Negative Experiences." In: S. Folkman (Ed.) *The Oxford Handbook of Stress, Health, and Coping*. New York: Oxford University Press.

Wilson, T. D., and D. T. Gilbert. 2003. "Affective Forecasting." *Advances in Experimental Social Psychology* 35: 345–411.

Chapter 7

Beck, A. T. 1999. *Prisoners of Hate: The Cognitive Basis of Anger, Hostility, and Violence*. New York: Harpercollins.

Beck, A. T., A. J. Rush, B. F. Shaw, and G. Emery. 1979. *Cognitive Therapy of Depression*. New York: Guilford.

DiGiuseppe, R., and R. C. Tafrate. 2007. *Understanding Anger Disorders*. New York: Oxford University Press.

Ellis, A., and R. A. Harper. 1975. *A New Guide to Rational Living*. Englewood Cliffs, N.J.: Prentice-Hall.

Epstein, N. B., and D. H. Baucom. 2002. *Enhanced Cognitive-Behavioral Therapy for Couples: A Contextual Approach*. Washington, DC: American Psychological Association.

Leahy, R. L. 2018. *Science and Practice in Cognitive Therapy: Foundations, Mechanisms, and Applications*. New York: Guilford Publications.

Chapter 8

Parker, A. M., W. B. De Bruin, and B. Fischhoff. 2007. "Maximizers versus Satisficers: Decision-Making Styles, Competence, and Outcomes." *Judgment and Decision Making* 2(6): 342.

Schwartz, B., A. Ward, J. Monterosso, S. Lyubomirsky, K. White, and D. R. Lehman. 2002. "Maximizing Versus Satisficing: Happiness Is a Matter of Choice." *Journal of Personality and Social Psychology* 83(5): 1,178–1,197. https://doi.org/10.1037/0022-3514.83.5.1178.

Chapter 10

Fairburn, C. G. 2013. *Overcoming Binge Eating: The Proven Program to Learn Why You Binge and How You Can Stop*. New York: Guilford Press.

Joiner, T. E., Jr., J. S. Brown, and J. Kistner (Eds.). 2006. *The Interpersonal, Cognitive, and Social Nature of Depression*. Mahwah, NJ: Erlbaum.

NIAAA. 2018. "Understanding Alcohol's Impact on Health." The National Institute on Alcohol Abuse and Alcoholism. Retrieved from: https://www.niaaa.nih.gov/publications/brochures-and-fact-sheets/understanding-alcohol-impact-health

Nolen-Hoeksema, S., L. E. Parker, and J. Larson. 1994. "Ruminative Coping with Depressed Mood Following Loss." *Journal of Personality and Social Psychology* 67: 92–104.

Papageorgiou, C., and A. Wells,. 2001a. "Metacognitive Beliefs About Rumination in Recurrent Major Depression." *Cognitive and Behavioral Practice* 8: 160–164.

Papageorgiou, C., and A. Wells. 2001b. "Positive Beliefs About Depressive Rumination: Development and Preliminary Validation of a Self-Report Scale." *Behavior Therapy* 32: 13–26.

Wells, A., and C. Papageorgiou. 2004. "Metacognitive Therapy for Depressive Rumination." In C. Papageorgiou and A. Wells (Eds.), *Depressive Rumination: Nature, Theory, and Treatment*. Chichester, UK: Wiley.

Robert L. Leahy, PhD, is author or editor of twenty-seven books, including *The Worry Cure*. He has led or been heavily involved with many national and international cognitive behavioral therapy (CBT) organizations. He writes a regular blog for *Psychology Today*, and has written for *HuffPost*. Leahy is an international speaker at conferences worldwide, and has been featured in print, radio, and television media such as *The New York Times*, *The Wall Street Journal*, *The Times*, *The Washington Post*, *20/20*, *The Early Show*, and more.

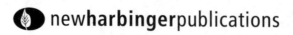

MORE BOOKS *from*
NEW HARBINGER PUBLICATIONS

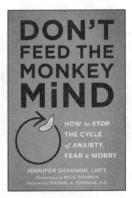
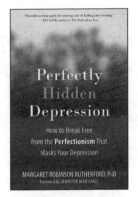

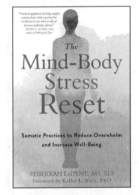
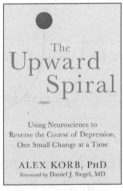
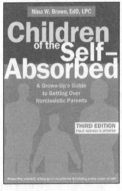
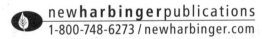

Register your **new harbinger** titles for additional benefits!

When you register your **new harbinger** title—purchased in any format, from any source—you get access to benefits like the following:

- Downloadable accessories like printable worksheets and extra content

- Instructional videos and audio files

- Information about updates, corrections, and new editions

Not every title has accessories, but we're adding new material all the time.

Access free accessories in 3 easy steps:

1. Sign in at NewHarbinger.com (or **register** to create an account).

2. Click on **register a book**. Search for your title and click the **register** button when it appears.

3. Click on the **book cover or title** to go to its details page. Click on **accessories** to view and access files.

That's all there is to it!

If you need help, visit:

NewHarbinger.com/accessories

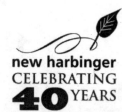

new harbinger
CELEBRATING
40 YEARS